T0259463

Substance Abuse in Office-Based Practice

Guest Editor

ROBERT MALLIN, MD

PRIMARY CARE:
CLINICS IN OFFICE PRACTICE

www.primarycare.theclinics.com

Consulting Editor
JOEL J. HEIDELBAUGH, MD

March 2011 • Volume 38 • Number 1

SAUNDERS an imprint of ELSEVIER, Inc.

W.B. SAUNDERS COMPANY
A Division of Elsevier Inc.

1600 John F. Kennedy Boulevard, Suite 1800 • Philadelphia, PA 19103-2899

http://www.theclinics.com

PRIMARY CARE: CLINICS IN OFFICE PRACTICE Volume 38, Number 1
March 2011 ISSN 0095-4543, ISBN-13: 978-1-4557-0496-5

Editor: Yonah Korngold

Primary Care: Clinics in Office Practice (ISSN: 0095–4543) is published quarterly by Elsevier Inc., 360 Park Avenue South, New York, NY 10010-1710. Months of issue are March, June, September, and December. Periodicals postage paid at New York, NY and additional mailing offices. Subscription prices are $203.00 per year (US individuals), $336.00 (US institutions), $101.00 (US students), $248.00 (Canadian individuals), $395.00 (Canadian institutions), $159.00 (Canadian students), $309.00 (international individuals), $395.00 (international institutions), and $159.00 (international students). Foreign air speed delivery is included in all *Clinics* subscription prices. All prices are subject to change without notice. POSTMASTER: Send address changes to *Primary Care: Clinics in Office Practice*, Elsevier Periodicals Customer Service, 11830 Westline Industrial Drive, St. Louis, MO 63146. Customer Service Health Sciences Division, Subscription Customer Service, 3251 Riverport Lane, Maryland Heights, MO 63043. **Customer Service: 1-800-654-2452 (U.S. and Canada); 314-447-8871 (outside U.S. and Canada). Fax: 314-447-8029. E-mail: journalscustomerservice-usa@elsevier.com (for print support); journalsonlinesupport-usa@elsevier.com (for online support).**

Reprints. For copies of 100 or more, of articles in this publication, please contact the Commercial Reprints Department, Elsevier Inc., 360 Park Avenue South, New York, NY 10010-1710. Tel. (212) 633-3812; Fax: (212) 482-1935; E-mail: reprints@elsevier.com.

Primary Care: Clinics in Office Practice is covered in *MEDLINE/PubMed (Index Medicus)* and *EMBASE/ Excerpta Medica, Current Contents/Clinical Medicine,* and *ISI/BIOMED.*

Printed and bound by CPI Group (UK) Ltd, Croydon, CR0 4YY

Transferred to Digital Print 2011

Contributors

CONSULTING EDITOR

JOEL J. HEIDELBAUGH, MD
Clinical Assistant Professor and Clerkship Director, Department of Family Medicine;
Clinical Assistant Professor, Department of Urology, University of Michigan Medical
School, Ann Arbor, Michigan

GUEST EDITOR

ROBERT MALLIN, MD
Professor, Family Medicine, Psychiatry and Behavioral Science, Medical University
of South Carolina, Charleston, South Carolina

AUTHORS

DANESH A. ALAM, MD
Associate Medical Director, Optum Health Behavioral Solutions, Schaumburg; Assistant
Professor of Clinical Psychiatry, University of Illinois at Chicago, Chicago; Central Dupage
Hospital, Winfield, Illinois

JOSEPH J. BENICH III, MD
Assistant Professor, Department of Family Medicine, Medical University of South Carolina,
Charleston, South Carolina

RICK BOTELHO, MD
Professor of Family Medicine & Nursing, University of Rochester, Rochester Center
to Improve Communication in Health Care, Building Relationships,
Eliminating Disparities, Rochester, New York

GARY D. CARR, MD, FAAFP, FASAM
Diplomate, American Board of Addiction Medicine; Medical Director, Professionals
Health Network, Inc, Hattiesburg, Mississippi; Past President Federation of State
Physician Health Programs, American Medical Association, Chicago, Illinois; Board
Registered Interventionist II, American Intervention Specialists, Lancaster,
Pennsylvania

DANIEL CICCARONE, MD, MPH
Associate Professor of Clinical Family and Community Medicine; Co-Director,
Foundations of Patient Care, Department of Family and Community Medicine,
University of California at San Francisco, San Francisco, California

D. TODD DETAR, DO
Clinical Professor, Department of Family Medicine, Medical University of South Carolina,
Charleston, South Carolina

BRETT ENGLE, PhD, LCSW
Assistant Professor, Barry University, Miami Shores, Florida

JOHN R. FREEDY, MD, PhD
Assistant Professor, Department of Family Medicine, Medical University of South Carolina, Charleston, South Carolina

SAMUEL N. GRIEF, MD, FCFP
Associate Professor in Clinical Family Medicine; Associate Professor, Department of Family Medicine; Medical Director, CampusCare, University of Illinois at Chicago, Chicago, Illinois

CHERYL HOLDER, MD
Associate Professor, Department of Humanities, Health and Society, Herbert Wertheim College of Medicine, Florida International University, Miami, Florida

ROBERT MALLIN, MD
Professor, Family Medicine; Psychiatry and Behavioral Science, Medical University of South Carolina, Charleston, South Carolina

JEANNE M. MANUBAY, MD
Assistant Clinical Professor of Medicine in Psychiatry, Division on Substance Abuse, New York State Psychiatric Institute; Assistant Attending Physician in Family Medicine, Departments of Family Medicine and Psychiatry, Columbia University, New York, New York

ANDREW MARTORANA, MD
Regional Medical Director, Optum Health Behavioral Solutions, Schaumburg, Illinois

JORGE CAMILO MORA, MD, MPH
Assistant Professor, Department of Humanities, Health & Society, Herbert Wertheim College of Medicine, Florida International University, Miami, Florida

CARRIE MUCHOW, EdM
Program Director, The Columbia University Buprenorphine Program, Department of Psychiatry, Columbia University, New York, New York

KATHERINE RYAN, BA
Psychology Intern, Department of Psychiatry and Behavioral Sciences, Medical University of South Carolina, Charleston, South Carolina

MARIA A. SULLIVAN, MD, PhD
Associate Professor of Psychiatry, Division on Substance Abuse, New York State Psychiatric Institute; Department of Psychiatry, Columbia University, New York, New York

Contents

Addiction is a chronic brain disease. Drug addiction manifests as a compulsive obsession to use a substance despite serious detrimental and sometimes irreversible consequences. Drug addiction is not the same as drug dependency because dependency may not manifest as an addictive behavior. This problem is fundamental to understanding the disease of addiction. This article discusses the neurobiology and genetics of drug addiction.

Alcohol dependency (alcoholism) has existed throughout recorded history. It remains a highly stigmatized illness, looked down on by society, the patients themselves, and the medical establishment. Science defines alcoholism as a primary progressive illness with a powerful genetic predisposition, highly amenable to intervention, evaluation, and treatment, and responsive to continuing care like other chronic illnesses. Society, led by an educated medical community, needs to revisit the disease of alcoholism, challenge its outdated assumptions and prejudices, and embark on a new course with the goals of positively affecting these patients, their families, and communities and improving the nation's health.

Nicotine dependence is a significant addiction with many health consequences. Consistent attempts and efforts at addressing this condition, guiding and advising afflicted patients using motivational techniques and the 5-A stepwise strategies, and instituting appropriate therapies will result in better health outcomes and less incidence of diseases. In pharmacotherapy, Nicotine replacement therapy and oral medications can be used alone or in combination with varying degrees of success.

The high prevalence of stimulant abuse and its harmful consequences make the screening, diagnosis, and referral for treatment of persons with stimulant abuse a top concern for primary care providers. Having a working knowledge of use patterns, clinical symptomatology, end-organ effects, and advances in treatment of stimulant abuse is essential. Although cocaine and amphetamine have different use patterns, duration of action, and so forth, the consequences of use are remarkably similar. Primary care is at the forefront of screening, brief risk reduction interventions, and diagnosis of medical sequelae, with referral to addiction specialist treatment when necessary.

Opioid dependence is becoming a more common problem in the United States that gives rise to many negative health and social consequences for both individuals and society as a whole. Opioid dependence presents a challenging issue for physicians to identify and treat. Understanding and managing withdrawal symptoms is often a necessary first step on the road to recovery for these patients. Long-term therapy options include detoxification, nonpharmacologic treatment plans, and maintenance replacement treatment with either methadone or buprenorphine. Physicians meeting necessary requirements have the option of implementing office-based opioid-assisted maintenance therapy.

The epidemic of prescription drug abuse has reached a critical level, which has received national attention. This article provides insight into the epidemiology of prescription drug abuse, explains regulatory issues, and provides guidelines for the assessment and management of pain, particularly with long-term opioid therapy. Using informed consent forms, treatment agreements, and risk documentation tools and regularly monitoring the 4 *A*'s help to educate patients and guide management based on treatment goals. By using universal precautions, and being aware of aberrant behaviors, physicians may feel more confident in identifying and addressing problematic behaviors.

This article presents an evidence-based approach to screening and case finding for alcohol use disorders in primary care. Problematic alcohol use by both adults and adolescents is considered. For clarity, this evidence-based presentation is divided into 6 sections: (1) epidemiology of alcohol use disorders, (2) associated health problems, (3) US Preventive Services Task Force screening recommendations, (4) screening/case finding instruments, (5) screening/case finding strategies, and (6) summary. This article reviews the state-of-the-art, evidence-based concepts and practices for screening and case finding for alcohol use disorders among adults and adolescents in primary care settings.

VISIT THE CLINICS ONLINE!

Access your subscription at:
www.theclinics.com

Foreword

Beyond Statistics, Motivating for Support

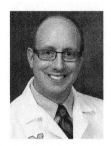

Joel J. Heidelbaugh, MD
Consulting Editor

Ah yes, the disheartening statistics about substance abuse. These numbers always baffle me, because with regard to either legal or illicit drugs, the prevalence of harmful substance abuse in America is always presented as either an increase or a decrease and neither case is looked upon favorably. When rates are reported as an increase, we become fearful and struggle to find acceptance in our current valiant efforts at improving patients' current lives and future outcomes; when rates are reported as a decrease, we shrug off the slight improvement and remain skeptical because we often don't see an appreciable change in our practices and in society at large.

What will provide an interesting angle to the problem of substance abuse in the coming years of healthcare reform are the issues of accountability and finance. This volume's guest editor, Dr Robert Mallin, an expert in family and addiction medicine, and his authors cite sobering literature supporting the inability of primary care physicians to appropriately diagnose and treat substance abuse disorders. Who is ultimately accountable for this? Is it the personal responsibility of individuals not to engage in cigarette smoking and alcohol and drug abuse in the first place, and to pay for their own rehabilitation and chronic disease management if one does become addicted? Or, is it the responsibility of health insurance companies and the taxpayers to fund rehabilitation programs? As more US citizens engage in illicit substance abuse, how can our exorbitantly expensive healthcare system possibly afford to offer adequate treatment to the masses?

Most clinicians would suggest a hybrid of both points of view, supporting increased provisions for support, treatment, and rehabilitation options for our patients. Yet, it still remains all too easy to "blame the system" for inadequate resources. Perhaps it took one of my patients to ask me to refer them to MTV's Celebrity Rehab (note, he wasn't a celebrity...) when his insurance wouldn't cover treatment for his heroin and cocaine addiction to realize that I was helpless in helping him. Undeniably, clinicians continue to report that they are poorly equipped with the skills to detect and treat

Prim Care Clin Office Pract 38 (2011) ix–x
doi:10.1016/j.pop.2010.12.004
0095-4543/11/$ – see front matter © 2011 Elsevier Inc. All rights reserved.

substance abuse and dependence. The concepts of motivational interviewing and teaching recovery theories to patients are often not included in medical student and primary care residency education, which greatly limits the role and comfortability of primary care clinicians to engage with patient substance abuse issues.

Moreover, patients increasingly deny that they are becoming addicted to prescription medications and often blame physicians not only for easy access, but also for not warning them of potential risk of dependence. Hydrocodone/APAP (Vicodin) accounted as the number 1 most costly generic drug in the US in 2009, with sales approaching $1.8 billion.[1] By way of comparison, OxyContin has now entered the top 10 in brand name prescription sales at number 8, accounting for over $3 billion in US sales in 2009.[2]

I would like to thank Dr Mallin and his authors for compiling a very detailed collection of reviews for this volume dedicated to addressing substance abuse in our patients. It is with these harrowing statistics, guidelines, and provisions, coupled with strategies to engage our patients to help themselves through goal setting and motivational interviewing, that we can all succeed in helping to achieve our patients in helping healthier lives.

Joel J. Heidelbaugh, MD
Departments of Family Medicine and Urology
University of Michigan Medical School
Ann Arbor, MI, USA

Ypsilanti Health Center
200 Arnet Street, Suite 200
Ypsilanti, MI 48198, USA

E-mail address:
jheidel@umich.edu

REFERENCES

1. Drug Topics. Pharmacy Facts and Figures. Available at: http://drugtopics. modernmedicine.com/drugtopics/data/articlestandard//drugtopics/252010/674976/ article.pdf. Accessed December 8, 2010.
2. Drug Topics. Pharmacy Facts and Figures. Available at: http://drugtopics. modernmedicine.com/drugtopics/data/articlestandard//drugtopics/252010/674961/ article.pdf. Accessed December 8, 2010.

Preface

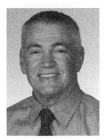

Robert Mallin, MD
Guest Editor

The prevalence of substance use disorders in primary care outpatients varies from 7 to 28%.[1,2] Drug use, including alcohol and tobacco, continues to be the greatest threat to our nation's health, causing well over 600,000 deaths yearly in the United States. Although the prevalence of drug use varies within populations, it remains significant for all groups seen in primary care medical practices.

Fifty percent of Americans currently drink alcohol. Twenty-three percent binge drink, defined as five or more drinks on at least one occasion in the 30 days prior to the survey. Seven percent are heavy drinkers, defined as binge drinking on 5 or more days in the past month. Twenty-four percent of Americans over 18 are current users of tobacco and 20.6% smoke cigarettes. Men (23.5%) were more likely than women (17.9%) to be current smokers. The prevalence of smoking was 31.1% among persons below the federal poverty level. For adults aged $\geq$25 years, the prevalence of smoking was 28.5% among persons with less than a high school diploma, compared with 5.6% among those with a graduate degree. Eight percent of the population aged 12 or older are current illicit drug users. Current drug use means use of an illicit drug during the month prior to the survey interview. Six percent are using marijuana, 1% using cocaine, and <1% using hallucinogens and heroin. Six percent of Americans abuse prescription medications.[3,4]

As with other chronic medical conditions, the best hope for prevention, detection, and treatment of substance use disorders begins with the primary care office visit. The primary care physician is uniquely situated to intervene in this area but often feels helpless to do so. Research reveals that primary care physicians in the United States perceive themselves as being less prepared to diagnose substance use disorders than other chronic conditions. They find it more difficult to discuss these topics with their patients and are more skeptical about the effectiveness of available treatments.[5] Despite these concerns, 88% of primary care physicians report that they routinely screen their patients for substance use problems and 82% refer their patients who screen positively for treatment. Further study reveals that although most of these physicians ask about alcohol consumption, less than 20% use a formal screening tool or ask follow-up questions important for diagnosing substance use disorders.[6]

Prim Care Clin Office Pract 38 (2011) xi–xii
doi:10.1016/j.pop.2010.12.003
0095-4543/11/$ – see front matter © 2011 Elsevier Inc. All rights reserved.

The purpose of this issue is to adequately arm the primary care provider with the knowledge and skills necessary to identify, treat, and/or refer patients with substance use disorders in the most effective means possible according to the best evidence available.

Robert Mallin, MD
Medical University of South Carolina
295 Calhoun Street, Room 126
Charleston, SC 29425, USA

E-mail address:
mallinr@musc.edu

REFERENCES

1. Fleming MF, Barry KL. The effectiveness of alcoholism screening in an ambulatory care setting. J Stud Alcohol 1991;52(1):33–6.
2. Miller PM, Thomas SE, Mallin R. Patient attitudes toward self-report and biomarker alcohol screening by primary care physicians. Alcohol Alcoholism 2006;41(3): 306–10.
3. Substance Abuse and Mental Health Services Administration. Results from the 2004 National Survey on Drug Use and Health: National Findings. Rockville (MD): (Office of Applied Studies, NSDUH Series H-28, DHHS Publication No. SMA 05–4062); 2005.
4. Substance Abuse and Mental Health Services Administration. Results from the 2003 National Survey on Drug Use and Health: National Findings. Rockville (MD): (Office of Applied Studies, NSDUH Series H-25, DHHS Publication No. SMA 04–3964); 2004.
5. Johnson TP, Booth AL, Johnson P. Physician beliefs about substance misuse and its treatment: findings from a U.S. survey of primary care practitioners. Subst Use Misuse 2005;40(8):1071–84.
6. Friedmann PD, McCullough D, Chin MH, et al. Screening and intervention for alcohol problems a national survey of primary care physicians and psychiatrists. J Gen Intern Med 2000;15(2):84–91.

Understanding the Disease of Addiction

D. Todd Detar, DO

KEYWORDS

• Drug addiction • Dopamine • Prefrontal cortex
• cAMP-responsive element binding

Addiction is a chronic brain disease. Drug addiction manifests as a compulsive obsession to use a substance despite serious detrimental and sometimes irreversible consequences. Drug addiction is not the same as drug dependency because dependency may not manifest as an addictive behavior. This problem is fundamental to understanding the disease of addiction. The area of the brain below the locus coeruleus (LC) and the median raphe region of the brain is where physical dependence occurs. The region above the LC in the ventral tegmental area (VTA) and nucleus accumbens (NA) is the heart of addiction neurocircuitry. Patients who are addictive are different from patients who have dependence, an important distinction to be made when choosing treatment options. Addiction has some stages in common; initiation, aberrant addictive behavior, and relapse, all associated with psychological denial. Once the brain becomes exposed to the substance ("I like the drug") changes occur in the normal brain circuitry, which is altered with repeated substance exposure, resulting in a very intense desire for the substance manifested as "I want the drug." Because the normal reward and adaptive behavior centers have been changed, the addictive behavior develops in the form of "I need the drug."[1] Exposure during brain development may result in greater brain changes as compared with after the brain is developed, causing more addiction during times of more risky behavior.[2] The brain changes cause a dysfunctional ability to render any control over the cravings or urge to use the substance, even at the expense of severe consequences, including death.[3] This repetitive corruption of motivational and learning circuitry by the substance causes abnormal changes in brain circuitry of rewarding and adaptive behavior centers, which leads to changes in brain structure that undermine voluntary control.[4,5] These areas of the brain are important for normal brain processes of motivation, reward, and inhibition in drug addiction. Drug addiction is a disease of the brain and the associated abnormal behavior is a result of dysfunctional brain tissue, as illustrated by imaging studies and aberrant behavior as seen with addiction.[3]

Department of Family Medicine, Medical University of South Carolina, 295 Calhoun Street, Charleston, SC 29425, USA
E-mail address: detardt@musc.edu

Prim Care Clin Office Pract 38 (2011) 1–7
doi:10.1016/j.pop.2010.11.001
0095-4543/11/$ – see front matter © 2011 Published by Elsevier Inc.
primarycare.theclinics.com

The neurobiological basis of addiction involves an understanding of brain pathways and neurochemistry in rewarding adaptive behaviors. Humans have adaptive, evolutionary systems in place, mediating acquisition of pleasurably rewarding behavior involved directly in the survival of the species, such as sex, food, and social interaction. We also avoid aversive events psychologically or physically to survive. Three main regions of the brain mediate adaptive behavior and the regulation of behavioral output. The NA, anterior in the mesolimbic system, mediates the positive reward behaviors and the amygdala (striatum) mediates the negative or fear-motivated behaviors. The prefrontal cortex (PFC) is involved in decision making by assigning stimuli to direct behavioral response (**Fig. 1**).[6]

Homeostasis of this neurobiological system uses internal motivation and emotional states combined with external incentive stimuli predicting reward, to determine the overall behavioral response by acquiring natural rewards or avoiding and decreasing painful states of consciousness.[7–9]

Drug addiction occurs as a result of neurobiological changes in areas of the brain that produce dopamine, such as the amygdala, medial forebrain bundle, VTA, anterior to the median raphe, and LC, which are related to areas affecting physical dependence (**Fig. 2**).[10]

Natural rewarding behaviors such as sex and food, and all drugs of abuse have a common neurotransmitter, dopamine, and have the ability to increase the levels of extracellular dopamine in the brain. Dopamine is increased in the NA, which is part of the common reward mesolimbic pathway from the VTA to the NA.[11]

The initial, acute "high" occurs because of enhanced dopamine transmission in the NA. Drugs of abuse increase dopamine in the NA to levels above what is normally seen for natural rewards, hijacking the reward system and corrupting the reward process.[12] A core feature of addiction is the persistence of aberrant behaviors despite tolerance

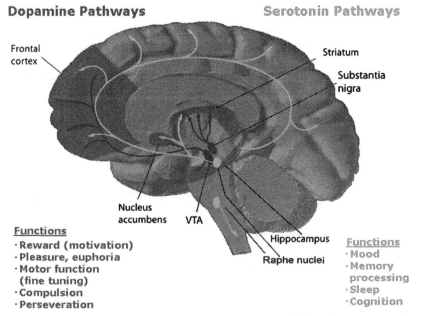

Dopamine Pathways

Serotonin Pathways

Frontal cortex

Striatum

Substantia nigra

Nucleus accumbens   VTA

Hippocampus

Raphe nuclei

Functions
- Reward (motivation)
- Pleasure, euphoria
- Motor function (fine tuning)
- Compulsion
- Perseveration

Functions
- Mood
- Memory processing
- Sleep
- Cognition

Fig. 1. Dopamine and serotonin pathways and functions. (*Data from* Kalivas PW. How do we determine which drug-induced neuroplastic changes are important? Nat Neurosci 2005; 8(11):1440–1.)

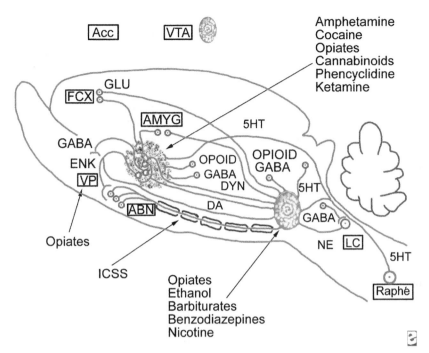

Fig. 2. The brain reward circuitry of the mammalian (laboratory rat) brain showing the sites at which various abusable substances appear to act to enhance brain reward and, thus, to induce drug-taking behavior and possibly drug craving. Acc, nucleus accumbens; AMYG, amygdala; DA, dopaminergic mesolimbic system; DYN, dynorphinergic outflow; ENK, enkephalinergic outflow; FCX, frontal cortex; GABA, GABAergic inhibitory fiber system; ICSS, component of reward circuitry preferentially activated by electrical intracranial self-stimulation; NF, noradrenergic fibers; VP, ventral pallidum. (*Data from* Gardner EL. Brain reward mechanisms. In: Lowinson JH, Ruiz P, Millman RP, et al, editors. Substance abuse. Baltimore (MD): William & Wilkins; 1997; and Gardner EL. Endocannabinoid signaling system and brain reward: emphasis on dopamine. Pharmacol Biochem Behav 2005;81(2):263–84.)

to positive effects of drugs over time. Addicts maintain use of the substance through negative reinforcement, partially to avoid negative states such as withdrawal.

Dopamine is increased either directly or indirectly. Direct increases occur by inhibition of reuptake at the neuron, or by stimulation of the release of dopamine by a stimulant such as cocaine or amphetamine. Indirect mechanisms that affect dopamine neuron firing occur when substances such as alcohol, opioids, nicotine, cannabis, or N-methyl-D-aspartic acid (NMDA) antagonists work on the mesolimbic system.[11]

Neurotransmitters including γ-aminobutyric acid (GABA), glutamate, acetylcholine, dopamine, serotonin, and endogenous opioid proteins have been studied in the effects of drugs of abuse. These neurotransmitters affect systems in conjunction with the mesolimbic dopamine system or independent pathways of reinforcement.[13] GABA interneurons modulate afferent inhibition of the release of dopamine in the VTA and NA.[14] The opioid system plays a role in modulation of the dopaminergic system with activation of mu-opioid receptors affecting dopamine levels, while also playing a role in reinforcing properties of alcohol and cannabis, and possibly playing a part in impulse control disorders.[15] The serotonin system has effects on the mesolimbic dopamine system, with changes in dopamine being seen.[16] The cholinergic system can stimulate dopamine release at the VTA to the NA. The nicotinic cholinergic receptors are implicated in the reinforcing properties of nicotine but also may affect opioid and cocaine reward reinforcement.[17]

The endocannaboinoid system mediates the reinforcing properties of cannabinoids (marijuana) that facilitate release of dopamine in the NA. The use of cannabinoid agonists and antagonists may be associated with blocking of reinforcing properties of cannabis, opioids, alcohol, cocaine, and nicotine in animal models.[12] Glutamate from the PFC stimulates dopamine release in the VTA and NA. The NMDA antagonists such as phencyclidine, ketamine, and dextromethorphan also exert reward-reinforcing properties.

Some argue that addiction fundamentally is a memory disorder whereby learning and memory become changed by drugs of abuse, resulting in maladaptive learning.[17]

In transition from abuse to dependence, all major drugs of abuse activate brain stress pathways, resulting in elevated adrenocorticotropic hormone, corticosterone, and corticotrophin releasing factor in the amygdala during withdrawal.[18] Some new treatment options with corticotrophin releasing factor 1 antagonist may represent a new class of antiaddictive treatment. As addiction progresses from the initial use to compulsive obsessive use, the neurobiology shifts from a dopamine-based behavioral system such as the initial rewarding aspects of drug use to a glutamate-based system relying still on dopamine. Conditioned responses, drug priming, and stress all cause relapse of the behavior without drug obsession.[19] As the move from abuse to dependence continues, habit response takes on new changes due to the dopamine in NA affecting the PFC and amygdala but not the NA, to start the process of relapse.[20] Dopamine release in the PFC and amygdala in the relapse state stimulates glutamate transmission between the PFC and amygdala and glutamate release in the pathway from the PFC to the NA core, constituting a "final common pathway" for drug-seeking obsession.[20] Glutamate dysregulation of the PFC and NA occurs; basal extracellular levels of glutamate in the NA are decreased in the addicted state with a decreased affinity for cystine-glutamate, nonsynaptic transportation. Consequently, agents that increase glutamate extracellularly may have some antiaddictive properties. PFC dysfunction in the orbitofrontal cortex and the anterior cingulate gyrus (where humans weigh up the pros and cons of engaging in particular behaviors normally) results in drug craving and impaired decision making. The major role of the anterior cingulate gyrus in inhibition sets patients up for loss of control and craving for a drug such as cocaine.[21]

GENETICS

Between 40% and 60% of the vulnerability to addiction is attributed to genetic factors.[22,23] Acute and chronic exposure to alcohol modulates function of the activity-dependent cyclic adenosine monophosphate–responsive element binding (CREB) protein in the brain, which may be associated with the development of alcohol addiction. Studying CREB has identified several important CREB-related genes, such as neuropeptide Y, brain-derived neurotrophic factor, activity-regulated cytoskeleton associated protein, and corticotrophin releasing factor, all playing a crucial role in the behavioral effects of alcohol as well as specific molecular changes to the neurobiology, underlying alcohol addiction, and a genetic predisposition to alcohol addiction.[24–27] CREB gene transcription factor may play a large part in the euphoric and dysphoric states in the development of alcohol addiction, playing a major role in changes in multiple areas of the brain including the NA, PFC, and cerebellum. Deficits of CREB in both the NA and amygdala, either innately or due to withdrawal after alcohol exposure, may promote alcohol intake. When CREB deficits are corrected, a decrease in alcohol consumption occurs and alcohol addiction is prevented. CREB function deficits may mediate the development of alcohol addiction by positive and negative affective states of alcohol addiction.[28]

Brain chromatin remodeling regulates gene expression via enzymatic restructuring of histone proteins and DNA without altering the primary genetic sequence.[29–31] Several key chromosomal regions in humans have been identified and linked to substance abuse, but only a few have polymorphisms that protect or predispose humans to drug addiction.[23] Polymorphisms in receptor genes mediating drug effects are associated with higher risk of addiction. An association has also been found between alcohol dependence and the genes for the type A GABA (GABA$_A$) receptors, specifically GABA receptor subunit α-2 (GABRA2) and GABA receptor subunit α-3 (GABRA3).[32–36]

ABSTINENCE-BASED REMISSION

Abstinence-based remission represents the most stable form of remission for most people recovering from alcohol addiction.[37] Controversy surrounds abstinence-based therapy and nonabstinence-based therapy.[38] Abstinence from all exposures of the substance currently makes good sense regarding relapse, whereby harm reduction programs such as methadone treatment or free needle distribution can alleviate the transmission rates of human immunodeficiency virus and hepatitis C infections.[39,40] It is clear that making the diagnosis of addiction rather than abuse is certainly a key factor in determination of the therapy.[41] The American Society of Addiction Medicine has multiple criteria for placement in different treatment options. From a neurobiological neuroanatomical point of view, abstinence-based therapy for the alcohol dependent makes clear sense.[10] The area of the brain below the LC and the median raphe region of the brain is where physical dependence occurs. The region above the LC in the VTA and NA is the heart of addiction neurocircuitry. Patients who are addictive are different from patients who have merely a physical dependence. For the alcohol abuser, harm reduction may play an important role in reducing the social and personal harm, but for a patient who is truly an addict, abstinence-based therapy will provide fewer exposures to manifest relapse while the brain is reconditioning through therapy. It would be like treating a patient whose illness is playing Russian roulette. Whether you take the gun away for abstinence therapy or just increase the number of guns with only one bullet for each, eventually you will have a problem.

REFERENCES

1. Kalivas PW, O'Brien C. Drug addiction as a pathology of staged neuroplasticity. Neuropsychopharmacology 2008;33(1):166–80.
2. Saraceno L, Munafo M, Heron J, et al. Genetic and non-genetic influences on the development of co-occurring alcohol problem use and internalizing symptomatology in adolescence: a review. Addiction 2009;104(7):1100–21.
3. Leshner AI. Addiction is a brain disease, and it matters. Science 1997;278(5335): 45–7.
4. Volkow ND, Fowler JS, Wang GJ. The addicted human brain: insights from imaging studies. J Clin Invest 2003;111(10):1444–51.
5. Fowler JS, Volkow ND, Kassed CA, et al. Imaging the addicted human brain. Sci Pract Perspect 2007;3(2):4–16.
6. Kalivas PW, Volkow ND. The neural basis of addiction: a pathology of motivation and choice. Am J Psychiatry 2005;162(8):1403–13.

7. Paulus MP. Neural basis of reward and craving—a homeostatic point of view. Dialogues Clin Neurosci 2007;9(4):379–87.
8. Hyman SE. Addiction: a disease of learning and memory. Am J Psychiatry 2005; 162(8):1414–22.
9. Hyman SE. The neurobiology of addiction: implications for voluntary control of behavior. Am J Bioeth 2007;7(1):8–11.
10. Gardner EL. Endocannabinoid signaling system and brain reward: emphasis on dopamine. Pharmacol Biochem Behav 2005;81(2):263–84.
11. Baler RD, Volkow ND. Drug addiction: the neurobiology of disrupted self-control. Trends Mol Med 2006;12(12):559–66.
12. Ross S, Peselow E. The neurobiology of addictive disorders. Clin Neuropharmacol 2009;32(5):269–76.
13. Koob GF, Volkow ND. Neurocircuitry of addiction. Neuropsychopharmacology 2010;35(1):217–38.
14. Heidbreder CA, Gardner EL, Xi ZX, et al. The role of central dopamine D3 receptors in drug addiction: a review of pharmacological evidence. Brain Res Brain Res Rev 2005;49(1):77–105.
15. Grant JE, Brewer JA, Potenza MN. The neurobiology of substance and behavioral addictions. CNS Spectr 2006;11(12):924–30.
16. Krystal JH, Petrakis IL, Krupitsky E, et al. NMDA receptor antagonism and the ethanol intoxication signal: from alcoholism risk to pharmacotherapy. Ann N Y Acad Sci 2003;1003:176–84.
17. Heidbreder C. Novel pharmacotherapeutic targets for the management of drug addiction. Eur J Pharmacol 2005;526(1–3):101–12.
18. Weiss F, Ciccocioppo R, Parsons LH, et al. Compulsive drug-seeking behavior and relapse. Neuroadaptation, stress, and conditioning factors. Ann N Y Acad Sci 2001;937:1–26.
19. Shaham Y, Hope BT. The role of neuroadaptations in relapse to drug seeking. Nat Neurosci 2005;8(11):1437–9.
20. Kalivas PW. Cocaine and amphetamine-like psychostimulants: neurocircuitry and glutamate neuroplasticity. Dialogues Clin Neurosci 2007;9(4):389–97.
21. Hester R, Garavan H. Executive dysfunction in cocaine addiction: evidence for discordant frontal, cingulate, and cerebellar activity. J Neurosci 2004;24(49):11017–22.
22. Uhl GR. Molecular genetics of substance abuse vulnerability: remarkable recent convergence of genome scan results. Ann N Y Acad Sci 2004;1025:1–13.
23. Uhl GR, Drgon T, Johnson C, et al. Addiction genetics and pleiotropic effects of common haplotypes that make polygenic contributions to vulnerability to substance dependence. J Neurogenet 2009;23(3):272–82.
24. Nestler EJ. Molecular mechanisms of drug addiction. Neuropharmacology 2004; 47(Suppl 1):24–32.
25. Pandey SC. The gene transcription factor cyclic AMP-responsive element binding protein: role in positive and negative affective states of alcohol addiction. Pharmacol Ther 2004;104(1):47–58.
26. Spanagel R. Alcoholism: a systems approach from molecular physiology to addictive behavior. Physiol Rev 2009;89(2):649–705.
27. Carlezon WA Jr, Duman RS, Nestler EJ. The many faces of CREB. Trends Neurosci 2005;28(8):436–45.
28. Moonat S, Starkman BG, Sakharkar A, et al. Neuroscience of alcoholism: molecular and cellular mechanisms. Cell Mol Life Sci 2010;67(1):73–88.
29. Jenuwein T, Allis CD. Translating the histone code. Science 2001;293(5532): 1074–80.

30. Impey S. A histone deacetylase regulates addiction. Neuron 2007;56(3):415–7.
31. Pandey SC, Ugale R, Zhang H, et al. Brain chromatin remodeling: a novel mechanism of alcoholism. J Neurosci 2008;28(14):3729–37.
32. Edenberg HJ, Dick DM, Xuei X, et al. Variations in GABRA2, encoding the alpha 2 subunit of the GABA(A) receptor, are associated with alcohol dependence and with brain oscillations. Am J Hum Genet 2004;74(4):705–14.
33. Edenberg HJ, Kranzler HR. The contribution of genetics to addiction therapy approaches. Pharmacol Ther 2005;108(1):86–93.
34. Dick DM, Edenberg HJ, Xuei X, et al. Association of GABRG3 with alcohol dependence. Alcohol Clin Exp Res 2004;28(1):4–9.
35. Enoch MA, Hodgkinson CA, Yuan Q, et al. The influence of GABRA2, childhood trauma, and their interaction on alcohol, heroin, and cocaine dependence. Biol Psychiatry 2010;67(1):20–7.
36. Zucker RA, Wong MM. Prevention for children of alcoholics and other high risk groups. Recent Dev Alcohol 2005;17:299–320.
37. Dawson DA, Goldstein RB, Grant BF. Rates and correlates of relapse among individuals in remission from DSM-IV alcohol dependence: a 3-year follow-up. Alcohol Clin Exp Res 2007;31(12):2036–45.
38. Flannery W, Farrell M. Harm reduction the key to managing problem drug users. Practitioner 2007;251(1694):99, 101–6.
39. Heilig M, Egli M, Crabbe JC, et al. Acute withdrawal, protracted abstinence and negative affect in alcoholism: are they linked? Addict Biol 2010;15(2):169–84.
40. Hughes JR. Measurement of the effects of abstinence from tobacco: a qualitative review. Psychol Addict Behav 2007;21(2):127–37.
41. Kornor H, Waal H. From opioid maintenance to abstinence: a literature review. Drug Alcohol Rev 2005;24(3):267–74.

Alcoholism: A Modern Look at an Ancient Illness

Gary D. Carr, MD[a,b,c],*

KEYWORDS

- Alcoholism • Addictive illness • Alcohol dependency
- Alcohol abuse • Addiction treatment

Alcohol is, perhaps, the oldest drug of abuse, second in incidence of use only to caffeine.[1,2] For most people alcohol use is enjoyable, unassociated with problems, and socially accepted. However, for about 10% of people, alcohol use progresses to alcohol abuse or alcohol dependency (alcoholism). This latter group suffers from a primary illness (a brain disease) with terrible morbidity and underreported mortality. Annually the United States bears an enormous and growing economic burden, spending conservatively $185 billion on lost productivity, health care, and associated societal ills.[1] When both drugs and alcohol among the estimated 10% of the population with addictive illness are considered, the cost to society is a staggering half a trillion dollars a year.[3,4]

The World Health Organization estimates that alcohol causes nearly 1.8 million deaths each year, with 76.3 million persons worldwide having diagnosable alcohol use disorders.[5] In the United States, excessive alcohol use is the third-leading lifestyle-related cause of death, responsible for up to 85,000 deaths annually.[6] Alcoholism is a family disease and results in untold suffering for the entire family. Nearly one-third of US adults drink enough to cause or place them at risk of adverse consequences. According to the Centers for Disease Control and Prevention, nearly 5% of the US population drink heavily, and 15% binge drink.[7] Much of the harm from alcohol comes from those who are not alcohol dependent, but who engage in excessive or hazardous drinking.[8]

Historically, we have attributed addictive illness, including alcoholism, to willful misconduct, character flaws, weak will, moral turpitude, or just bad people. Science does not support these outdated stereotypes. In 1956, the American Medical Association declared alcoholism an illness.[9] Hampered by prejudice, misinformation, and an

The authors have no funding support to disclose.
[a] Professionals Health Network, Inc, 5192 Old Highway 11, Suite 1, Hattiesburg, MS 39402, USA
[b] Federation of State Physician Health Programs, American Medical Association, 515 North State Street - Room 8584, Chicago, IL 60654, USA
[c] American Intervention Specialists, 313 West Liberty Street, Suite 129, Lancaster, PA, USA
* Professionals Health Network, Inc, 5192 Old Highway 11 Suite 1, Hattiesburg, MS 39402.
E-mail address: Docgcarr@aol.com

Prim Care Clin Office Pract 38 (2011) 9–21
doi:10.1016/j.pop.2010.11.002   primarycare.theclinics.com

0095-4543/11/$ – see front matter © 2011 Elsevier Inc. All rights reserved.

outdated sense of hopelessness at our supposed inability to effect meaningful intervention, the medical community has been slow to respond. Even today, most medical students and residents complete training without benefit of a rudimentary working knowledge of addictive illness; an illness they will see in their office almost daily for the rest of their careers.

Addiction is a disease of the patient's reward system, which alters behavioral drives that are under limited conscious control. Decision making is damaged such that abstinence is no longer simply a matter of choice. Gastfriend[10] dubs addictive illness "a brain disease that subverts self-preservation."

Evidence-based studies indicate that proper diagnosis, evaluation, treatment, and monitoring work. Perhaps the best example of success may be the experience of state physician health programs. In a recent study, 904 consecutively admitted physicians from 16 states followed with substance use disorder including alcoholism were monitored for an average of 7.2 years and showed only a 22% relapse rate throughout the period. After further intervention for those who did relapse, more than 90% of the sample were abstinent at monitoring after 7.2 years.[11,12] There are sentinel lessons in these data for the medical community and the general population. Addictive illness can be easily diagnosed and effectively treated and lives can be saved to the benefit of the patient, their families, their community, and society.

PATHOPHYSIOLOGY

Alcohol is a water-soluble molecule that is rapidly absorbed into the bloodstream from the stomach, small intestine, and colon and metabolized primarily in the liver by the actions of alcohol dehydrogenase (ADH) and mixed function enzymes. ADH converts alcohol to acetaldehyde, which is subsequently converted to acetate by the actions of acetaldehyde dehydrogenase (ALDH). Metabolism follows zero-order kinetics and alcohol is metabolized at a rate of about 28 g (1 ounce) every 3 hours.[1]

All areas of the brain are affected by alcohol, which shares some common pathways with benzodiazepines, barbiturates, and opiates. Excessive use of alcohol influences several neurochemical systems in the brain, including the γ-aminobutyric acid (GABA), glutamate, opiate, and, perhaps most importantly, the dopamine system. Dopamine neurons originate in the ventral tegmental area and project to discrete areas of the forebrain, including the nucleus accumbens, olfactory tubercle, frontal cortex, amygdala, and the septal area. These areas are involved in translating emotion into action through processing reward, pleasure, and the assignment of salience to important environmental stimuli. The brain of the alcoholic is changed in both structure and function. There is strong evidence to suggest that drugs of abuse, including alcohol, that activate the reward structures in the brain induce lasting changes in behavior that reflect changes in neuron physiology and biochemistry.[13] These changes can be seen on brain positron emission tomography (PET) scans of alcoholics but not of social drinkers.[1,14–16]

ALCOHOL ABUSE AND DEPENDENCY

Approximately two-thirds of all American adults drink an alcoholic beverage during the course of a year. It is estimated that 20% to 36% of patients in primary care practices drink excessively.[17] Alcohol use disorders, including alcohol abuse (**Box 1**) and dependence (**Box 2**), affect 7% to 8% of Americans at any given time,[14] or about 21 to 25 million adults. The National Institute on Alcohol Abuse and Alcoholism (NIAAA) recommends that men younger than 65 years drink no more than 4 drinks on an occasion or 14 in a week. For women of any age and men more than 65 years no more than

---

Box 1
Alcohol abuse

Alcohol abuse is defined as a maladaptive pattern of alcohol use leading to clinically significant impairment or distress, as manifested by 1 (or more) of the following, occurring within a 12-month period:

1. Alcohol prevents fulfillment of major role obligations (eg, home, work, or school)

2. Recurrent use of alcohol in physically hazardous situations

3. Recurrent alcohol-related legal problems

4. Continued use of alcohol in the face of social or interpersonal problems

5. Does not meet and has not met criteria for alcohol dependency

Data from Frances A. Substance related disorders. In: Diagnostic and statistical manual of mental disorders. 4th edition, text revision (DSM-IV-TR). Arlington (VA): American Psychiatric Association; 2000. p. 197, 198, 212–22.

---

3 drinks on an occasion or 7 drinks per week are recommended. More than this is considered excessive.

The research makes 1 statement that is clearly true: alcoholism is a primary, chronic brain disease. It is an independent disorder characterized by a craving for alcohol: a dependence, or addiction. Those with or without the illness may misuse the substance causing problems and various societal ills. Understanding that many of these people have an illness (alcoholism) does much to sharpen research and help dispel stigma from this major chronic disorder. The sine qua non of alcohol dependence (and addictive illness generally) is loss of control, such as the inability to cut down, stop, or predict outcome once drinking starts despite adverse consequences.

Alcohol is, arguably, the number 1 drug of abuse among young people, rivaling marijuana and, more recently, opiates. Adolescents who expose their developing brain to alcohol before age 15 years are 4 times more likely to develop alcohol dependence than those who begin drinking at age 21 years.[17]

Box 2
Alcohol dependency

Alcohol dependency (alcoholism) is defined as a maladaptive pattern of alcohol use leading to clinically significant impairment or distress, as manifest by 3 or more of the following, occurring at any time in the same 12-month period:

1. Tolerance

2. Withdrawal

3. Use of more alcohol or use for a longer time than intended

4. Unsuccessful efforts or desire to cut down or control alcohol use

5. A great amount of time is spent getting alcohol, using alcohol, or recovering from use

6. Alcohol-associated decrease in important social, occupational, or recreational activities

7. Continued use in the face of persistent or recurrent physical or psychological problems

Data from Frances A. Substance related disorders. In: Diagnostic and statistical manual of mental disorders. 4th edition, text revision (DSM-IV-TR). Arlington (VA): American Psychiatric Association; 2000. p. 197, 198, 212–22.

Addiction vulnerability is related to genetic influences, environmental conditions, complex personality traits, stress responses, and comorbid issues, including self-medication of undiagnosed psychiatric illness, family of origin issues, history of sexual abuse and other trauma, and poor coping skills.

DIAGNOSIS

Health care professionals can quickly master various brief screening instruments. Perhaps the simplest is the CAGE (cut down, annoyed, guilty, eye-opener) questions. This quick screen takes only seconds and has been found to be 82% sensitive and 79% specific for problematic alcohol consumption. Other easily obtained quick screening instruments include the Alcohol Use Disorders Identification Test, or the Michigan Alcoholism Screening Test.[18–20] These and other screening instruments are readily available online through the American Academy of Family Practice, the American Society of Addiction Medicine, the NIAAA, and related sites.

The DSM-IV criteria for alcohol abuse and dependency[21] are undergoing needed review and update. Less emphasis needs to be attributed to tolerance and withdrawal, which are only physiologic manifestations of use, and more emphasis should be directed toward negative consequences, craving, and loss of control.

It is particularly important that health care professionals learn to recognize and correctly diagnose alcohol abuse and dependency to better aid this population. A study of care quality in primary care determined that patients with alcohol dependence received only 11% of recommended care.[22]

DENIAL

Denial, a hallmark of addictive illness, makes early intervention challenging and treatment and recovery difficult. Denial is not lessened by education or training and, to the contrary, may contribute to a more highly developed denial mechanism.[23] The level of denial present can often be astounding and requires recognition and the assistance of both patient and family as they progress through the stages of recognition and change. Not infrequently, the patient remains in such denial of their illness that formal intervention using trained professionals or involvement of the legal system for commitment may become necessary for the patient's survival.

GENETICS

Genetics play a major role in expression and type of alcoholism (**Box 3**). Animal studies, adoption studies, twin studies, studies on sons of alcoholics, and the Collaborative Study on the Genetics of Alcoholism (COGA), among others, are clear and convincing.[1,24]

Sons of alcoholics consistently rated alcohol effects less than nonalcoholics, showed less objective ataxia, and were less likely to experience hangovers than sons of nonalcoholics.[25] These signs could be predictive of future risk for developing alcoholism in this population.

Humans and rodents share most of their genes and respond to alcohol in similar ways. Many rat and mouse strains have been developed to study alcohol and other drugs. Animal models may provide clues that accelerate the search for alcohol-related genes.[1]

Adoption and twin studies show substantial heritability in both men and women, and there seem to be multiple genes at play. Ample research exists to say that although a significant portion of an individual's genetic makeup (50%–60%) determines risk

Box 3
Type 1 and type 2 alcoholics
Type 1
75% of alcoholics
Low alcohol seeking and violence
Psychological dependence with fear and guilt
Low novelty seeking, high harm avoidance
Requires genetic makeup and environmental factors
Onset after age 25 years
Type 2
25% of alcoholics
Infrequent fear and guilt
High novelty seeking, low harm avoidance
Primarily genetic
Onset before age 25 years

for alcoholism, nonbiologic factors (environmental) also play a role and to different degrees depending on the type of alcohol dependency involved.

COGA is a 6-center study exploring the genetics of alcoholism. The task of the study is difficult because alcoholism is considered to be a polygenic disorder that is related to different genes, each of which contributes only a portion of the vulnerability. COGA scientists have identified several hot spots (areas of potential linkage to alcohol dependence) on chromosomes 1, 2, and 7 and possible protective factors by linkage on chromosome 4.

Genetics may also help explain the higher incidence of psychiatric comorbidity in the alcoholic population. For instance Wang and colleagues[26] note that the cholinergic muscarinic 2 receptor has been associated with the function of memory and cognition. Variations in the gene responsible for the production of this receptor predisposed to both alcohol dependence and major depression. COGA scientists believe there is a link to alcoholism and depression on chromosome 1. Luo and colleagues[27] note specific alleles, genotypes, haplotypes, and diplotypes significantly associated with risk for either alcohol dependence or affective disorders.

ACUTE INTOXICATION AND ALCOHOL WITHDRAWAL

As seen on college campuses each year, acute intoxication may be life threatening. The most important principle in management is to prevent severe respiratory depression and to protect the airway to prevent aspiration.[28] Absorption of alcohol occurs quickly; therefore induction of emesis and gastric lavage is not indicated unless the exposure is treated within 30 to 60 minutes. There is no effective alcohol antagonist. Agitation is typically managed with reassurance. In more severe cases, a short-acting, rapid-onset benzodiazepine (eg, lorazepam) alone, or in combination with a neuroleptic agent such as haloperidol, can be useful.

For alcoholics, withdrawal can manifest 6 to 24 hours after the last drink. Early symptoms include anxiety, sleep disturbances, vivid dreams, anorexia, nausea, and headache. Physical signs include tachycardia, increased blood pressure, hyperactive reflexes, sweating, tremor, and hyperthermia. Withdrawal seizures are most likely within 48 hours of cessation. Alcohol withdrawal delirium, or delirium tremens, typically begins 48 to 72 hours after the last drink. Mortality is believed to be 1% to 5%. A symptom-triggered response using benzodiazepines is effective. Thiamine, folic acid, and magnesium are typically depleted and should be replaced.

Management of acute intoxication and withdrawal may be a necessary first step but does nothing to address the critically important underlying addictive illness. Directing the patient to appropriate treatment is critical and must not be overlooked.

Physical dependence is an important factor in continued drinking by an alcoholic because cessation of alcohol drinking induces unpleasant and occasionally life-threatening symptoms of withdrawal. In human alcoholics, tolerance to the sedative and even lethal effects of alcohol can be profound. Physical dependence is defined as the occurrence of symptoms that appear after the cessation of alcohol drinking. These symptoms include both physical and psychological components and enhanced craving.

HEALTH CONSEQUENCES

Moderate alcohol use (2 drinks for men, 1 for women) may be helpful by decreasing risk of coronary heart disease. However, its misuse, abuse, and dependency have many well-recognized health consequences for the individual and implications for society.[29] Fibrosis and cirrhosis of the liver may be among the most serious consequences of alcohol abuse, accounting for about 50% of deaths from liver disease. From a cardiovascular standpoint, alcohol can lead to hypertension, increased risk of coronary artery disease and stroke, cardiomyopathy with heart failure, and atrial fibrillation/other arrhythmias.[30]

Neurologically, alcohol damages neurons diffusely but especially the limbic system, diencephalon, and the frontal cerebral cortex. It is estimated that alcohol-induced dementia in the United States is second only to Alzheimer disease. Alcohol interferes with absorption of nutrients and vitamins and is associated with several serious neurologic sleep disturbances, and psychoses such as Wernicke and Korsakoff psychoses.

Alcohol can interfere with the endocrine system, impairing reproductive development and functioning as well as libido in both women and men. In premenopausal women, chronic heavy drinking can contribute to problems with the menstrual cycle, early menopause, increased risk of spontaneous abortions, and increased risk for breast cancer. It can alter the secretion of growth hormone, resulting in numerous metabolic and endocrine changes. For the pregnant woman alcohol is responsible for fetal alcohol syndrome and alcohol-related neurodevelopmental disorders.[31]

Alcohol affects the immune system by altering the function, regulation, and distribution of lymphoid cells, with increased susceptibility to infectious disease and cancer. There is a 3- to 5-fold increased risk of postoperative infection, prolonged stays in the intensive care unit, and longer hospital stays for those with alcohol use disorder. Nosocomial pneumonia, particularly *Klebsiella pneumoniae*, is the most frequent. Pneumonia affects 38% of alcoholic patients postoperatively compared with 7% of nonalcoholics. Alcoholics are also seen to have more postoperative bleeding complications and are twice as likely to require secondary surgeries.[32]

Alcohol misuse, abuse, and dependency are responsible for up to 40% to 50% of cases seen in trauma and burn units. Motor vehicle accidents, falls, fires, and drownings cause more than 75% of deaths from alcohol-associated unintentional injuries (NIAAA reports).[33] Alcohol is a significant contributing factor in most fatal prescription drug overdoses.[34] There is a strong relationship between alcohol and various types of violence, including homicides, suicides, and spousal abuse. More than 60% of persons who committed homicides had been drinking (NIAAA reports). Patients presenting in the emergency room (ER) who had received violent injuries were twice as likely to have consumed alcohol as were patients whose injuries were unrelated to violence (NIAAA reports). Alcohol use is correlated with high-risk sexual behaviors and the attendant increased incidence of infection with the human immunodeficiency virus and hepatitis B and C.

In addition to health consequences, those with alcohol use disorders show more neglect of work and family, and costs to society associated with police, courts, jails, use of medical services, social programs, and unemployment.

TREATMENT

Appropriate care requires intervention, detoxification, acute treatment, and long-term management. Only about 13% of persons with alcohol dependency receive specialized addiction treatment, and only 24% seek any kind of help.[35] The peak age for those entering treatment is 35 to 45 years, although these patients met criteria for alcohol dependency a decade earlier. Intervention and treatment are effective for adolescents as well as adults, although somewhat less so for the former.[14,36–38]

Most alcohol/addiction treatment centers are based on the Minnesota treatment model,[39] which is derived from Alcoholics Anonymous (AA). Treatment involves education, psychotherapy groups, AA/Narcotics Anonymous, individual therapy, and treatment of co-occurring psychiatric illness. Competent continuing care after treatment should include regular follow-up with knowledgeable professionals, as with all other chronic illnesses. I encourage a contract between the patient and their primary care or addiction medicine specialist. Medication proved to aid abstinence should be considered.

Behavioral therapies (with or without pharmacotherapies) include AA, group therapy, motivational enhancement therapy, cognitive-behavioral therapy, vocational counseling, and family therapy. Behavior-modification techniques emphasizing self-diagnosis, self-responsibility, and development of coping skills and techniques that patients can use to recognize and manage situations that may trigger craving and relapse are important.

Comorbid psychiatric illness is frequently seen with addictive illness.[40] Examples include major depression, anxiety disorders, and posttraumatic stress disorder. When present, both alcoholism and psychiatric illness are primary, and both require concurrent treatment if recovery is to be sustained.

Family involvement is important in constructing a support system for all involved. Family members who understand the illness of addiction, avoid enabling behaviors, and attend their own recovery needs improve outcomes.[41,42]

PHARMACOTHERAPY

Research continues regarding development of new drugs to aid recovery from alcoholism. Few effective pharmacotherapies are available, although there are medications with significant usefulness with which health care professionals should be familiar. Medication should be prescribed only within the context of a global approach to care that includes psychosocial support.

Alcohol use while taking disulfiram (Antabuse) causes nausea, vomiting, and facial flushing. These effects occur via inhibition of ALDH, resulting in a buildup of acetaldehyde. Although disulfiram has been used since 1949, studies in 1986 questioned its efficacy because alcoholics discontinue the drug and drink.[43] Disulfiram may be particularly useful in some groups who can be carefully monitored for compliance.

Naltrexone (oral Revia or long-acting injectable Vivitrol) is an agent that blocks opioid receptors, particularly the μ-opioid receptor, leading to decreased levels of dopamine in the nucleus accumbens. Naltrexone seems to help with environmental cues, the associated craving, and alcohol use. It is generally well tolerated (**Box 4**). Naltrexone lessens the stimulant effect of alcohol and increases its sedative and other negative effects.[14,44] There is evidence of the usefulness of combination disulfiram and naltrexone.[14,45,46]

Several studies have shown acamprosate (Campral) may reduce cravings as well as the frequency and intensity of relapse to alcohol. Its effectiveness is not supported in other studies. Acamprosate affects the GABA and glutamate neurotransmission center, particularly the latter; however, the underlying mechanism of action is poorly understood.[21,44]

Topiramate (Topamax) showed some usefulness in decreasing drinking among those who had not yet stopped drinking in that they tended to drink less often and less per drinking occasion.

Selective serotonin reuptake inhibitors (SSRIs), particularly fluoxetine (Prozac) and citalopram (Celexa), have been studied by multiple investigators, who noted the class tendency to reduce alcohol consumption in mice. The effect with human subjects seems to be transient and inconsistent. Notwithstanding, many alcoholics have co-occurring mood disorders, and these studies may allow us to feel more comfortable using this drug class when indicated.

Box 4
Naltrexone: common side effects

Abdominal pain/cramps

Diarrhea

Nausea/vomiting

Fatigue

Headache

Depression

Irritability

Sleep disturbance

Ejaculation dysfunction

Anxiety

Arthralgia

Chills

Constipation

Dizziness

Impotence

Myalgia

Rash

Note: Must be abstinent from opioids before use to avoid precipitating withdrawal.

Most patients feel much improved after detoxification from alcohol but a subset have a protracted postwithdrawal syndrome (protracted withdrawal) manifested by anxiety, insomnia, and general distress, which can last weeks or months. This syndrome may best be addressed through the assistance of an addiction medicine physician. SSRIs are believed safer than tricyclic antidepressants in this situation. Some believe the judicious use of benzodiazepines such as chlordiazepoxide may have less abuse potential than others in the class and support their judicious use. Other addiction professionals do not believe benzodiazepines have a place in the treatment of the recovering alcoholic.

RELAPSE

Relapse in alcoholism/addictive illness is interesting in that the health care community mistakenly views it as failure, unlike the relapse in other chronic illnesses such as hypertension, asthma, and diabetes. Relapse is not failure; rather it is a common, although not inevitable, symptom of this chronic brain disease. Cellular adaptation and reinforcement, both positive and negative, acting in concert, determine an individual's long-term or chronic craving for alcohol that characterizes dependence. Some adaptive changes may be permanent and are hypothesized to produce the persistent sense of discomfort during abstinence that can trigger relapse. Understanding relapse is critical to effectively treating alcohol dependence.

Powerful neurophysiologic mechanisms are at play that contribute to distorted thinking in the recovering alcoholic. These functional changes are well documented in PET examinations of the limbic and control brain regions, further confirming that addiction is a disease with definable, reproducible, anatomic, and biochemical brain alterations.[4,34]

Risk factors for relapse can include environmental cues, any mood-altering substance, and stress. Domino and colleagues[47] noted a higher instance of relapse in health care professionals who (1) had a family history of addictive illness, (2) had a history of both psychiatric illness and addiction to major opioids, and (3) had a coexisting psychiatric disorder.

Perhaps the most exciting data regarding the possibilities for sustained remission come from Domino and colleagues' study[47] and a more recent study by McClellan and colleagues[11,12] involving recovering physicians. McLellan and colleagues documented total abstinence rates exceeding 78% without relapse at 7.2 years and more than 90% in sustained recovery when those with brief relapse and additional treatment are considered.

PREVENTION

Prevention is preferable to treatment. Prevention is challenging and there are cultural, societal, and economic issues at play.[48] An educated health care community adept at identifying and addressing addictive illness can make a difference. Men who engaged in excessive drinking responded to intervention of only 1 to 4 sessions administered by a physician, nurse, or psychologist. They reduced weekly alcohol consumption 1 year later with fewer ER visits and fewer alcohol-related injuries.[8] School-based programs, linked to other community activities, show promise. Evidence indicates intervening with individuals who have been injured as a result of their drinking may prove a useful clinical strategy, reducing subsequent drinking and readmission for traumatic injuries, as well as drinking and driving, traffic violations, alcohol-related injuries, and alcohol-related problems among 18- and 19-year-olds.[49,50]

In view of the global burden of alcoholism, much needs to be done. Some recommend an international health policy, in the form of a Framework Convention on Alcohol Control, to counterbalance the global conditions promoting alcohol-related harm and to support and encourage international action.[51]

Evidence exists that increased price, decreased availability, and less alcohol advertising are cost-effective strategies to reduce harm. Education of the public as to the extent of the problem and effective paths forward is needed.[52]

Addiction screening, brief interventions, diagnosis, medication management, and referrals to appropriate resources must become a mandated component at all curricular levels of training programs for health care providers.

SUMMARY

Alcoholism and other drug dependencies are primary illnesses, and effective intervention, treatment, and sustained recovery should be the expected result of our efforts as health care professionals. As has been pointed out in this article, we have much work to do.

The medical education system continues to produce health care professionals without the tools needed to recognize and effectively intervene with addictive illness. This system, which strives to provide its students with the tools they need and the confidence to use them, lags well behind the curve regarding addictive illness. Too often, the medical education system itself is part of the culture of neglect, hopelessness, indifference, and stigmatization. Our patients with addictive illness may not expect more, but they deserve better. Few endeavors hold the promise for our nation's health as does a long-overdue examination and revamping of the approach of this system to addictive illness. Understanding addictive illness as the brain disease science shows it to be makes ongoing stigmatization of its sufferers antiquated and its continuation an impediment to meaningful solutions. The time has come to move beyond the moral model of addiction; it lacks usefulness and validity and is counterproductive.

The Wellstone-Domenici Mental Health Parity Act requiring parity for our patients with mental and addictive illness passed into law and is in the implementation stage. We must demand this law have teeth and that our patients have affordable access to evidence-based treatments that have been proved to save lives.

Addiction professionals, managed care plans, medical educators, legislators, and society demand and deserve evidence-based data. The research explosion of the last 3 decades must be funded and supported. Just as importantly, we must ensure that the insights gained through research are efficiently translated into effective patient care.

Studies demonstrate the cost benefit to society when people with addictive illness receive treatment. Indeed the CALDATA (California Drug and Alcohol Treatment Assessment) study[53] and the Northwest Professional Consortium Report[54] indicate consistent and marked improvement across multiple indicators . CALDATA reported that for each $1 spent on education, prevention, and treatment, $7 is saved in services.[34,53] The approach of government to addictive illness has been heavily weighted toward interdiction, incarceration, and expensive social programs. Yet, of the half a trillion dollars the United States spends each year, only about 1.5% goes to education, prevention, and treatment combined. A fundamental examination of our national strategy with reallocation of our resources is desperately needed. Drug courts around the country have proved highly effective. These and similar contingency-management innovations should be heartily supported. Government must also come to terms with the fact that our nation's "War on Drugs" is an abject failure. The interdiction of drugs does nothing to address a growing demand spurred by addictive illness. Where demand exists, supply inevitably follows. Meanwhile, our expensive prisons are filled to overflowing with our citizens, many of whom are there because of the consequences of untreated addictive illness. Interdiction and incarceration are not treatment and recovery, therefore the cycle continues.

As we consider alcoholism and other addictive illnesses in the early twenty-first century, there are many great challenges yet to be faced. However, progress is being made and there is hope that much more can be done. Alcoholism and other addictive illness are easily diagnosed. Effective treatments exist and models for effective disease management have been reported. Research continues to unravel the mysteries of this complex illness, and new drug treatments are emerging that show promise. There is good cause to believe that further study will continue to yield even more effective, science-based strategies for prevention and treatment. There is reason to hope that the burden of alcohol abuse and alcoholism on individuals, families, communities, and nations will be dramatically improved. Health care professionals will know we have made great progress on this journey when our patients feel able to come to us, unburdened by shame or fear, and say, "I'm an alcoholic and I need your help."

REFERENCES

1. Woodward J. The pharmacology of alcohol. In: Graham A, Terry K, Mayo-Smith MF, et al, editors. Principles of addiction medicine. 3rd edition. Chevy Chase (MD): American Society of Addiction Medicine; 2003. p. 101–18.
2. Berge K, Seppala M, Lanier W. The anesthesiology community's approach to opioid and anesthetic-abusing personnel. Anesthesiology 2008;109:762–4.
3. National Institute on Drug Abuse. NIDA InfoFacts: treatment approaches for drug addiction. Washington, DC: US Deprttment of Health and Human Services; 2009. (Sept): all.
4. National Institute on Drug Abuse. NIDA InfoFacts: treatment approaches for drug addiction. Washington, DC: US Department of Health and Human Services; 2008. (June): all.
5. World Health Organization. Global status report on alcohol 2004. Available at: http://www.who.int/substance_abuse/publications/global_status_report_2004_overview.pdf. Accessed September 30, 2008.
6. Mokdad A, Marks J, Stroup D, et al. Actual causes of death in the United States, 2000. JAMA 2004;291(10):1238–45.
7. Centers for Disease Control and Prevention. Alcohol and public health. Available at: http://www.cdc.gov/alcohol/. Accessed September 30, 2008.
8. Kaner E, Beyer F, Dickinson H, et al. Effectiveness of brief alcohol interventions in primary care populations. Cochrane Database Syst Rev 2007;2:CD004148.
9. Report of the Board of Trustees. JAMA 1956;162:750.
10. Gastfriend D. Physician substance abuse and recovery: what does it mean for physicians–and everyone else? JAMA 2005;293:1513–5.
11. Dupont R, McLellan T, Carr G, et al. How are addicted physicians treated? A national survey of physician health programs. J Subst Abuse Treat 2009;37:1–7.
12. McLellan T, Skipper G, Campbell, et al. Five year outcomes in a cohort study of physicians treated for substance use disorders in the United States. BMJ 2008; 337:a2038.
13. Mohn A, Yao W, Caron M. Genetic and genomic approaches to reward and addiction. Neuropharmacology 2004;47:101–10.

14. Anton R. Naltrexone for the management of alcohol dependence. N Engl J Med 2008;359(7):715–21.
15. Kobb G, Roberts A, Schulteis G, et al. Neurocircuitry targets in ethanol reward and dependence. Alcohol Clin Exp Res 1998;22:3–9.
16. Fiellin D, Carrigton R, O'Connor P. New therapies for alcohol problems: application to primary care. Am J Med 2000;108:227–37.
17. Grant B, Harford T, Dawson D, et al. Prevalence of DSM-IV alcohol abuse and dependence: United States, 1992. Alcohol Health Res World 1994;18(3):243–8.
18. Buchsbaum D, Buchanan R, Centor R, et al. Screening for alcohol abuse using CAGE scores and likelihood ratios. Ann Intern Med 1991;115(10):774–7.
19. Babor T, Higgins-Biddle J, Saunders J, et al. The Alcohol Use Disorders Identification Test: guidelines for use in primary care. 2nd edition. Geneva (Switzerland): World Health Organization; 2001. Available at: http://whqlibdoc.who.int/hq/2001/WHO_MSD_MSB_01.61.pdf. Accessed September 30, 2008.
20. Willenbring M. National Institute on Alcohol Abuse and Alcoholism. Helping patients who drink too much: a clinician's guide and related professional support resources. Available at: http://www.niaaa.nih.gov/Publications/EducationTrainingMaterials/guide.htm. Accessed September 30, 2008.
21. Frances A. Substance related disorders. In: Diagnostic and statistical manual of mental disorders. text revision (DSM-IV-TR). 4th edition. Arlington (VA): American Psychiatric Association; 2000. p. 197, 198, 212–22.
22. McGlynn E, Asch S, Adams J, et al. The quality of health care delivered to adults in the United States. N Engl J Med 2003;348(26):2635–45.
23. White R, Kitlowiski E. Physicians in recovery. Md Med J 1998;37:183–9.
24. Tapper A, McKinney S, Nashmi R, et al. Nicotine activation of alpha 4 receptors: sufficient for reward, tolerance, and sensitization. Science 2004;306:1029–32.
25. Svhuckit M, Smith T. An 8-year follow-up of 450 sons of alcoholics and controls. Arch Gen Psychiatry 1996;53:202–10.
26. Wang J, Hindrichs A, Stock H, et al. Evidence of common and specific genetic effects: association of the muscarinic acetylcholine receptor M2 (CHRM2) gene with alcohol dependence and major depressive syndrome. Hum Mol Genet 2004;13:1903–11.
27. Luo X, Kranzler H, Zuo L, et al. CHRM2 gene predisposes to alcohol dependence, drug dependence and affective disorders: results from an extended case-control structured association study. Hum Mol Genet 2005;14:2421–34.
28. Mayo-Smith M. Management of alcohol intoxication and withdrawal. In: Graham A, Terry K, Mayo-Smith MF, et al, editors. Principles of addiction medicine. 3rd edition. Chevy Chase (MD): American Society of Addiction Medicine Inc; 2003. p. 621–31.
29. Gordis E. Understanding alcoholism: insights from the research. In: Graham A, Terry K, Mayo-Smith MF, et al, editors. Principles of addiction medicine. 3rd edition. Chevy Chase (MD): American Society of Addiction Medicine; 2003. p. 33–45.
30. Krishnamoorthy S, Lip G, Lane D. Alcohol and illicit drug use as precipitants of atrial fibrillation in young adults: a case series and literature review. Am J Med 2009;22(9):851–6, e3.
31. Janzen L, Nanson J, Block G. Neuropsychological evaluation of preschoolers with fetal alcohol syndrome. Neurotoxicol Teratol 1995;17(3):273–9.
32. Lau A, Dossow V, Sander M, et al. Alcohol use disorders and preoperative immune dysfunction. Anesth Analg 2009;108:916–20.
33. Lowenfels A, Miller T. Alcohol and trauma. Ann Emerg Med 1984;13:1056–60.
34. Hall P, Hawkinberry H, Moyers-Scott P. Prescription drug abuse & addiction: past, present and future: the paradigm for an epidemic. W V Med J 2010;106(4):24–30.

35. Dawson D, Grant B, Stinson F, et al. Recovery from DSM-IV alcohol dependence: United States, 2001–2002. Addiction 2005;100(3):281–92.
36. Moss H, Chen C, Yi H. Subtypes of alcohol dependence in a nationally representative sample. Drug Alcohol Depend 2007;91(2–3):149–58.
37. Tripodi S, Bender K, Litschge C, et al. Interventions for reducing adolescent alcohol abuse. Arch Pediatr Adolesc Med 2010;164(1):85–91.
38. Brown S, McGue M, Maggs J, et al. A developmental perspective on alcohol and youths 16 to 20 years of age. Pediatrics 2008;121:S290–310.
39. Kirn T. Advances in understanding of alcoholism initiate evolution in treatment programs. JAMA 1986;256:1405–12.
40. Bryson E, Jeffrey S. Addiction and substance abuse in anesthesiology. Anesthesiology 2008;109:905–17.
41. O'Connor P, Spickard A. Physician impairment by substance abuse. Med Clin North Am 1997;81:1037–52.
42. Glanter M, Casteneda R, Franco H. Group therapy and self-help groups. In: Frances R, Miller S, editors. Clinical textbook of addictive disorders. New York: Guilford Press; 1991. p. 431–51.
43. Fuller R, Branchey L, Brightwell D, et al. Disulfiram treatment of alcoholism. A Veteran's Administration cooperative study. JAMA 1986;256:1449–55.
44. Kranzler H, Jaffe J. Pharmacologic interventions for alcoholism. In: Graham A, Terry K, Mayo-Smith MF, et al, editors. Principles of addiction medicine. 3rd edition. Chevy Chase (MD): American Society of Addiction Medicine Inc; 2003. p. 701–19.
45. Haley T. Disulfiram (tetraethylthioperoxydicarbonic diamide): a reappraisal of its toxicity and therapeutic application. Drug Metab Rev 1979;9:319–55.
46. Johnson B, Rosenthal N, Capece J, et al. Topiramate for treating alcohol dependence: a randomized controlled trial. JAMA 2007;298(14):1641–51.
47. Domino KB, Hornbein TF, Polissar NL, et al. Risk factors for relapse in health care professionals with substance use disorders. JAMA 2005;293:1453–60.
48. Hankes L, Bissell L. Health professionals. In: Lowinson J, Ruiz P, Millman R, editors. Substance abuse: a comprehensive textbook. Baltimore (MD): Williams & Wilkins; 1992. p. 897–908.
49. Gentileoo L, Rivara F, Donovan D, et al. Alcohol interventions in a trauma center as a means of reducing the risk of injury recurrence. Ann Surg 1999;230(4): 473–83.
50. Monti P, Colby S, Barnett N, et al. Brief intervention for harm reduction with alcohol-positive older adolescents in a hospital emergency department. J Consult Clin Psychol 1999;67(6):989–94.
51. Cassell S, Thamarangsi T. Reducing harm from alcohol: call to action. Lancet 2009;373(9682):2173–6.
52. Anderson P, Dan C, Fuhr D. Alcohol and Global Health 2. Effectiveness and cost-effectiveness of policies and programs to reduce the harm caused by alcohol. Lancet 2009;373:2234–46.
53. CALDATA data. Evaluating recovery services: the California Drug and Alcohol Treatment Assessment, report to State of California Dept of Alcohol and Drug Programs. Available at: http://aspe.hhs.gov/hsp/caldrug/caldata.htm. Accessed November 27, 2010.
54. Finigan M. Societal outcomes and cost savings of drug and alcohol treatment in the state of Oregon. Prepared for Office of Alcohol and Drug Abuse Programs Oregon Department of Human Resources by Northwest Professionals Consortium; February 20, 1996.

Nicotine Dependence: Health Consequences, Smoking Cessation Therapies, and Pharmacotherapy

Samuel N. Grief, MD, FCFP[a,b,*]

KEYWORDS

• Nicotine dependence • Smoking cessation therapies
• Tobacco • Nicotine replacement therapy

Cigarette and other tobacco products contain nicotine. Nicotine is a highly addictive substance, thought by some to be the most addictive drug available.[1] Nicotine addiction and tobacco use are responsible for more disease and death than any other medical condition in the United States and are rapidly becoming the No. 1 cause of death worldwide.[2] At present, there are about 1.3 billion smokers living in the world; most (84%) live in developing countries.[2] If current trends continue, tobacco will kill 10 million people each year by 2020.[2]

Tobacco use has been cited as the chief avoidable cause of illness and death in the society and accounts for more than 435,000 deaths each year in the United States.[3] Smoking is a known cause of multiple cancers, heart disease, stroke, complications of pregnancy, chronic obstructive pulmonary disease (COPD), and many other diseases.[3] In addition, recent research has documented the substantial health dangers of involuntary exposure to tobacco smoke.[4] Despite these health dangers and the public awareness of those dangers, tobacco use remains surprisingly prevalent. Recent estimates are that about 21% of adult Americans smoke, representing approximately 45 million current adult smokers.[5] Moreover, tobacco use remains a pediatric disease.[6] Each day, about 4000 youth aged 12 to 17 years smoke their first cigarette, and about 1200 children and adolescents become daily cigarette smokers.[7]

This work is unfunded.

[a] Department of Family Medicine, University of Illinois at Chicago, 1919 West Taylor Street, Suite 159, Chicago, IL 60612, USA

[b] CampusCare, University of Illinois at Chicago, 820 South Wood Street, W310 CSN, Chicago, IL 60612, USA

* Department of Family Medicine, University of Illinois at Chicago, 1919 West Taylor Street, Suite 159, Chicago, IL 60612.

E-mail address: sgrief@uic.edu

Prim Care Clin Office Pract 38 (2011) 23–39
doi:10.1016/j.pop.2010.11.003   **primarycare.theclinics.com**
0095-4543/11/$ – see front matter © 2011 Elsevier Inc. All rights reserved.

As a result, new generations of Americans are at risk for the extraordinarily harmful consequences of tobacco use.

Tobacco use exacts a heavy cost to society and individuals. Smoking-attributable health care expenditures are estimated at $96 billion per year in direct medical expenses and $97 billion in lost productivity.[8] If all smokers covered by state Medicaid programs quit, the annual savings to Medicaid would be $9.7 billion after 5 years.[9]

Research investigating why people smoke has shown that smoking behavior is multifaceted. Factors influencing smoking initiation differ from those of smoking behavior maintenance. Nicotine dependence, genetic factors, and psychosocial factors influence maintenance of smoking behavior.[10]

Nicotine is a potent psychoactive drug, often inducing euphoria; serves as a reinforcer of its use; and leads to strong and overwhelming withdrawal symptoms in its absence.[10] As an addictive drug, nicotine has 2 very potent issues: it is a stimulant and it is also a depressant. Therefore, lighting up and inhaling a cigarette can both perk one up in the morning and help de-stress at the end of a busy or stressful workday. These associations of pleasure and reward have helped nicotine and tobacco use infiltrate themselves into the lives of millions upon millions of people and they continue to do so.

Nicotine influences the levels of many neurochemical substances and hormones. Nicotine increases the levels of endorphins, and corticosteroid levels increase in proportion to plasma nicotine concentration. Nicotine alters the bioavailability of dopamine and serotonin and acts on brain reward mechanisms, indirectly through endogenous opioid activity and directly through dopaminergic pathways.[10]

The association between smoking and mood and psychiatric disorders is indisputable.[11] A lifetime history of major depression is more than twice as common in people who smoke compared with people who do not smoke.[10] Between 72% and 90% of schizophrenic patients smoke cigarettes compared with 24% of the general population.[12] Nicotine administration has been found to improve perception and attention to moving stimuli in patients with schizophrenia. Not surprisingly, nicotine replacement treatment has been shown to improve memory in schizophrenic patients.[13] Smoking is also associated with psychosis in bipolar affective disorder.[14]

HEALTH CONSEQUENCES OF SMOKING AND NICOTINE ADDICTION

Despite the many prior reports on the topic and the high level of public knowledge in the United States of the adverse effects of smoking in general, tobacco use remains the leading preventable cause of disease and death in the United States. An increasingly disturbing situation of widespread organ damage in active smokers is emerging, likely reflecting the systemic distribution of tobacco smoke components and their high level of toxicity (**Box 1**).[15]

Cancer

It is estimated that approximately one-third of all cancer deaths worldwide are attributable to tobacco use.[16] Cigarette smoke contains more than 4000 chemicals and upwards of 60 known carcinogens, including tobacco-specific nitrosamines and polycyclic aromatic hydrocarbons.[17] The longer and more frequently a person smokes, the more likely a tobacco-related cancer will develop. For this reason, addiction is a strong indirect contributor to other diseases, in that it promotes high-level and persistent exposure to cancer-causing agents.

Because most tobacco users are cigarette smokers who inhale smoke into the lungs, active smoking and exposure to environmental tobacco smoke are believed

---

Box 1
Health consequences of smoking

Cancers

- Lung cancer
- Oral cancer
- Laryngeal cancer
- Esophageal cancer
- Pancreatic cancer
- Bladder cancer

Cardiovascular diseases

- Coronary artery disease
- Stroke
- Hypertension
- Peripheral vascular disease

Lung diseases

- COPD
- Exacerbation of asthma

Pregnancy-related complications

- Low birth weight
- Preterm births
- Perinatal deaths

Effects on children

- Sudden infant death syndrome
- Otitis media (ear infections)
- Asthma
- Bronchitis and pneumonia
- Wheezing and lower respiratory illness

Miscellaneous

- Periodontal (gum) disease
- Cataracts
- Macular degeneration
- Premature aging of the skin
- Erectile dysfunction
- Infertility

---

to account for 90% of all cases of lung cancer. A marked increase in lung cancer incidence has occurred in all countries where smoking has increased. Secondhand smoke (SHS) has also been found to be a direct cause of lung cancer, resulting in 3000 cases of lung cancer in the United States annually.[18] In the United States, lung cancer is responsible for more deaths than any other kind of cancer and since the mid-1980s, it has killed more women each year than breast cancer.[18] It is estimated that 85% of all cases of lung cancer could be prevented if smoking of ciga-rettes is stopped.[18] However, exposure to carcinogens is not limited to the respiratory system. Smoking is a major cause of bladder cancer, pancreatic cancer, laryngeal cancer, oral cancer, and esophageal cancer. Quitting smoking decreases the cancer risk both immediately and in the long term, although not to the level of someone who has never smoked. Smokeless tobacco users, meanwhile, repeatedly expose the oral mucosa to toxins and have a substantially increased risk of getting head and neck cancers.[19]

SHS is a known carcinogen and is responsible for more than just lung cancer. Every year, SHS causes an estimated 46,000 nonsmokers living with smokers to die from heart disease, causes 300,000 lung infections in children younger than 18 months, and increases the number and severity of asthma attacks in 1 million children with asthma.[20]

Lung Disease

Smokers suffer from many respiratory diseases other than lung cancer. One such disease is COPD, which is one of the major causes of debilitation and eventual death in cigarette smokers. More than 80% of those diagnosed with COPD are smokers, and most of these people die prematurely, with a greater number of women dying from COPD than men.[21] Avoidance of smoking is the most important preventive measure. Smoking cessation is imperative for patients with COPD, and physicians must persuade afflicted patients that it is never too late to quit smoking.[22,23] Active smoking and exposure to environmental tobacco smoke are also responsible for increases in other respiratory ailments, such as pneumonia, bronchitis, the common cold, and influenza. Smokers who contract these ailments take longer than nonsmokers to recover. Children are especially susceptible to the effects of environmental tobacco smoke. When raised in a household where children are regularly exposed to environ-mental tobacco smoke, they are more likely to suffer from asthma, ear infections, respiratory infections, and chronic cough.[18,24]

Heart Disease

Smoking has long been recognized as a major risk factor in cardiovascular disease, the risk being greater the more one smokes.[25] Globally, there are regional and cultural differences in the incidence of smoking-related cardiovascular disease. For example, among the 3 cigarettes smoked in the world today, 1 is smoked in China where smoking rates have increased steadily since the 1970s.[26] As a result, about 63% of adult men smoke (as opposed to 4% of adult women), yet cardiovascular disease makes up a much smaller percentage of smoking-related deaths than in the United States and Europe, where it accounts for approximately 30% to 40% of all tobacco-caused deaths.[27] After quitting, a smoker's risk for cardiovascular disease decreases faster than the risk for lung cancer, with reductions in risk evident within 1 year of cessation.

Effects on Pregnancy

Smoking remains the single most important preventable cause of poor birth outcome. Smoking is responsible for 20% low-birth-weight deliveries, 8% preterm births, and 5% perinatal deaths.[28] When a pregnant woman smokes, some toxins from the smoke can be passed to the fetus. These toxins can later affect an infant's lung development and function.[29] Babies of smoking women are more likely to be born prematurely, to have a low birth weight, and to have slower initial growth.[28] Smoking cessation within the first trimester lowers these health risks to a level comparable to those of people who have never smoked. There is a 2-fold increased rate of sudden infant death syndrome associated with maternal cigarette smoking.[30]

Smoking and Other Diseases

Smoking is a significant risk factor for the development of periodontal (gum) diseases. Risk calculations suggested that 40% of chronic periodontitis cases may be attributed to smoking.[31] People who smoke cigarettes are at increased risk for developing cataracts. Tobacco smoking is also one of the preventable risk factors for age-related macular degeneration.[32] Smoking cigarettes ages skin faster than anything else apart from sun damage.[33] There is a growing body of literature supporting the association between smoking and erectile dysfunction.[34] Smoking directly affects male and female fertility, with a higher rate of miscarriage among female smokers.[35,36]

SMOKING CESSATION THERAPIES AND GUIDELINES

Smoking may begin as a voluntary habit but eventually, it becomes an addiction. As Mark Twain famously put it, "Quitting smoking is easy. I've done it a thousand times." Health professionals can contribute powerfully to motivate their patients to attempt and sustain cessation by offering encouragement, advice, and assistance. For patients who are not yet ready to attempt quitting, such advice can move them further toward that point. A willingness to help and provide assistance is important in motivating cigarette smokers in attempting to quit. The reassurance that a knowledgeable health professional stands ready to offer guidance and support is immensely beneficial to individuals addicted to nicotine.

According to the US Preventive Services Task Force guidelines, clinicians should ask all adults about use of tobacco products and provide cessation interventions to current users.[37] The guideline engages a "5-A" approach to counseling, including

- Ask about tobacco use.
- Advise to quit through personalized messages.
- Assess willingness to quit.
- Assist with quitting.
- Arrange follow-up care and support.

Brief behavioral counseling (ie, <10 minutes) and pharmacotherapy are effective alone, although they are most effective when used together.[37]

The Task Force also advises clinicians to inquire all pregnant women, regardless of age, about tobacco use. Those who smoke should receive pregnancy-tailored counseling supplemented with self-help materials.

Understanding the benefits and limitations of the available medications provides an important foundation for such a successful smoking cessation program.

The smoking history, level of addiction, and the health status of the patient should be assessed. After the assessment, it is recommended to intervene with education and advice (**Box 2**).

In the following section, the strategies advocated to help patients achieve a nonsmoking status are outlined in more detail. Not surprisingly, the 5-A approach has been endorsed by many commercial health insurance plans.[38]

Ask: find out if patient smokes or has recently quit.

Advise: goal is to either present compelling evidence about the importance of quitting and/or encourage recent quitters to continue abstinence. Message must be strong, clear, and relevant to specific patient's concerns.

Identify and assess: does the patient currently smoke? If no, has the patient smoked in the past? If yes, assist with cessation maintenance (see step 4) and determine if the patient is willing to quit (also known as readiness to

---

Box 2
Smoking cessation strategies for the administering physicians

Strategy 1: Ask

    Systematically identify all tobacco users at every visit

Strategy 2: Advise

    Strongly urge all smokers to quit

Strategy 3: Identify

    Find smokers willing to quit

Strategy 4: Assist

    Aid the patient in quitting

    Help patient with a quit plan

    Encourage pharmacologic therapies

    Provide supplementary materials

Strategy 5: Arrange

    Schedule follow-up contact

---

change). If not willing to quit, provide motivational materials and counseling. If yes, provide appropriate cessation techniques (see step 4). Further steps in assessing patient's reasons for not taking action include

1. If the patient is resistant, find out why patient does not want to quit.
2. Emphasize risks of smoking.
3. Point out the rewards of quitting.
4. Discuss roadblocks and ways to overcome them.

Assist: find common ground with patients. Appropriate use of motivational interviewing (MI) technique has proved useful in smoking cessation efforts. MI is a directive patient-centered style of counseling, designed to help people explore and resolve ambivalence about behavior change.[39] A more direct approach may also be highly effective. Providing direct feedback to patients during the counseling session often prompts an action plan to form. Helpful aspects of counseling include providing problem-solving guidance for smokers to develop a plan to quit and to overcome common barriers to quitting as well as providing social support within and outside treatment. For example, uncover why people smoke and educate regarding coping strategies. Are they addicted to nicotine? Try drinking lots of water. Do they derive enjoyment? Do something else enjoyable. Are they susceptible to common triggers like smoking after eating? Have a breath mint. Are there social situations or peer pressure to smoke? Avoid situations where there is smoke. Do patients encounter roadblocks, such as friends who smoke? Talk on the phone instead of talking in person. Is the patient just not motivated, stating something to the effect of "I don't really want to quit but I know I should?" If so, help them identify personal reasons to quit. Try sharing some tangible short-term rewards, such as clothes and breath will smell better, cough will go away, more money for incidental expenses, sense of smell will improve. See **Box 3** for a summary of how to create a smoking cessation plan.

Arrange for follow-up: for patient who has remained smoke-free, offer congratulations. For patient who has relapsed, return to "Assist" step in the 5-A approach.

> **Box 3**
> **Creating a smoking cessation plan**
>
> Step 1: Identify why people smoke, common triggers, and major roadblocks
>
> Step 2: Identify rewards
>
> Step 3: Establish a quit date
>
> Step 4: Identify cessation method and coping strategies
>
> Step 5: Provide resources. For a patient who has remained smoke free, offer congratulations. For a patient who has relapsed, return to "Assist" step in the 5-A approach. What was the trigger? When did the relapse occur? What was going on in the patient's life at the time of relapse? Did the patient have a support person there? What techniques did the patient try to help work through the craving? Would the patient like to set another quit date?

PHARMACOTHERAPY FOR NICOTINE DEPENDENCE
Nicotine Replacement Therapy

The most widely studied and used pharmacotherapy for managing nicotine dependence and withdrawal is therapeutic use of nicotine-containing medications.[40] Nicotine medications make it easier to abstain from tobacco by replacing, at least partially, the nicotine formerly obtained from tobacco and thereby providing nicotine-mediated neuropharmacologic effects.

There are at least 3 major mechanisms of action by which nicotine replacement therapy (NRT) medications support smoking cessation efforts.[41] First, the medications may reduce either general withdrawal symptoms or at least prominent ones, thus enabling people to function while they learn to live without cigarettes. Second, the medications may also reduce the reinforcing effects of tobacco-delivered nicotine. Third, nicotine medications may provide some effects for which the patient previously relied on cigarettes, such as sustaining desirable mood and attention states, making it easier to handle stressful or boring situations, and managing hunger and body weight gain.

All the approved nicotine replacement medications have been determined by the US Food and Drug Administration (FDA) to be safe and effective aids to smoking cessation. It should be noted that not all reinforcing effects of tobacco are solely attributable to nicotine. Over time, the various sensory stimuli accompanying cigarettes and cigarette smoking become effective at both triggering and relieving tobacco cravings. For example, denicotinized cigarettes have been shown to temporarily reduce tobacco craving and some withdrawal symptoms in abstinent smokers, although it has been long known that they are unsatisfactory substitutes for nicotine-containing cigarettes in the long run.[42]

Conversely, although even intravenous nicotine can partially substitute for smoking, reduce spontaneous smoking, and reduce urges to smoke, sensory stimuli can be as important if not more important in the short run. For example, in one study comparing the effects of intravenous nicotine, smoking regular cigarettes, and smoking denicotinized cigarettes, administration of intravenous nicotine caused a small suppression of ad libitum smoking behavior, whereas denicotinized smoke produced a significantly larger reduction, showing that short-term satiation is more dependent on the presentation of smoke than delivery of nicotine per se.[43] However, denicotinized smoke alone did not have as much effect as puffs from the usual brands of cigarettes. Further, a meta-analysis of studies of denicotinized cigarettes found that ratings of smoking derived from denicotinized cigarettes varied with level of tobacco dependence, suggesting that sensory factors may be more important to highly dependent smokers than less dependent smokers.[44] Furthermore, nicotine replacement medications such as nicotine gum and patch can substantially reduce most physiologic and cognitive withdrawal symptoms while tobacco cravings persist (albeit typically at lower levels). A clinical implication of such observations is that nicotine replacement medications should not be viewed as stand-alone medications that make people stop smoking. They reduce withdrawal and dependence, but it may take many months if not years for some people to be able to comfortably manage their cravings in a world filled with tobacco-associated stimuli. NRT is most effective when used in conjunction with behavioral and other types of nonpharmacologic cessation interventions.[41] Reassurance and guidance from health professionals combined with medication can be critical for some people to achieve and sustain abstinence.

Currently Approved Products

There are 6 types of nicotine replacement products in the global market. These include several brands and types of nicotine transdermal patch systems that deliver nicotine through the skin, nicotine nasal spray, and several products that deliver nicotine through the oral mucosa, such as, gum, lozenge, sublingual tablet, and vapor inhaler.

A Cochrane meta-analysis of 132 trials in which any type of NRT and a placebo or non-NRT control group was included showed improved successful smoking cessation with all commercially available forms of NRT (gum, transdermal patch, nasal spray, inhaler, and sublingual tablets/lozenges). Overall, NRT products increase the rate of quitting by 50% to 70% and seem to be independent of any additional support.[45]

Nicotine patches are applied once per day. The other products allow the smoker to self-administer a dose of nicotine on an as-needed basis. Combination therapy using both patches and as-needed nicotine products is becoming increasingly the standard of care of NRT (see section on Combination Therapy).[46]

The following sections describe the dosing, instructions for use, expected adverse events, and notable characteristics of each formulation. It should be noted that there are some adverse events that are common to all NRT products, including dizziness, nausea, and headache. Therefore, the following sections discuss only adverse events that are specific to that delivery form. See **Tables 1** and **2** for a summary of the pharmacotherapy for nicotine dependence and the side effects of smoking cessation medications.

Transdermal Nicotine Patches

The patch should be applied to a clean, dry, nonhairy area on the trunk or upper arm. Remove the patch from the package, peel off the protective strip, and immediately apply it to the site. Press firmly for 10 to 20 seconds to make sure the patch stays in place. Be sure the edges are held firmly to the skin. Wash your hands after applying the patch. Different brands of nicotine patches vary in the length of time the patch is left on the skin (eg, for 24 hours [all day and night] vs 16 hours [all day]). Remove the patch carefully and dispose of it properly, and keep away from children. Apply each new patch to a different area to prevent skin irritation. Do not suddenly stop using this medication because withdrawal symptoms may develop. Gradually decreasing the dose is most commonly recommended.

Smokers who use 10 or less cigarettes per day are instructed to begin with the medium dose of the patch. For some products, progressively lower doses can be used to provide weaning over a period of several weeks or longer to enable gradual adjustment to lower nicotine levels and ultimately to a nicotine-free state.

Table 1
Pharmacotherapy for nicotine dependence

	Dosing	Instructions
Over-the-Counter Medication		
Nicotine Gum	Use 2-mg (<20 cigarettes/d) and 4-mg (>20 cigarettes/d) pieces on a regular schedule or as needed. Up to 24 pieces may be used daily. Wean after 6 wk and again at 10 wk	Chew the gum slowly until flavor is tasted. Then park the gum between the cheek and gum to permit absorption through the oral mucosa. Repeat when taste subsides for about 30 min. Do not take with food or drink. Use for up to 12 wk
Nicotine Lozenge	2-mg lozenge for lighter smokers, and 4-mg lozenge for heavier smokers. Same dosing and weaning as gum	Suck on lozenge until it dissolves. Do not bite, chew, or swallow. Do not take with food or Drink. Use for up to 12 wk
Nicotine Patch	Use 1 patch daily. Nicoderm CQ (GlaxoSmithKline, London, UK) is a 24-h patch that comes in 3 doses for tapering. Recommended dosing is 21 mg for 4 wk, 14 mg for 2 wk, and 7 mg for 2 wk. Nicotine (Nicotrol) is a 16-h patch that also comes in 3 doses. Use 15-mg dose initially. Use for up to 8 wk	Every morning, place a fresh patch on a relatively hairless area of the skin between the waist and neck. Remove at bedtime if sleep disruption occurs. Use HC cream for minor skin reactions. Use for up to 8 wk
Sublingual Tablet[a]	Hold under the tongue, where the nicotine is absorbed sublingually. The levels of nicotine obtained by use of the 2-mg tablet and 2-mg nicotine gum are similar	Use for up to 12 wk, then taper
Prescription Medication		
Nicotine Inhaler (Nicotrol)	Puff as needed. One cartridge delivers 4 mg of nicotine in the course of 80 inhalations (about 20 min). Typical dosing is 6–16 cartridges/d. Taper use in the last 6–12 wk of use	Do not take with food or drink Use for up to 6 mo
Nicotine Nasal Spray (Nicotrol NS)	A dose is 1 spray in each nostril (1 mg total nicotine). Initial treatment is 1–2 doses per h, as needed. Typical dosing is 8–40 doses/d. Each bottle contains 100 doses	Tilt the head back slightly during administration; do not sniff, inhale, or swallow. Use for up to 6 mo
Bupropion SR (Zyban, Wellbutrin)	Take 150 mg for first 3 d, 300 mg after day 3	Begin 1–2 wk before quit date. Limit alcohol use. Use for up to 6 mo
Varenicline (Chanitx)	Take 0.5 mg daily for 3 d, then 0.5 mg daily for 4 d, and then 1 mg twice daily for up to 12 wk	Begin 1 wk before quit date. Use for up to 24 wk

Abbreviations: HC, hydrocortisone; SR, sustained release.
[a] Not available in the United States as of 2010.
Adapted from Fiore MC, Bailey WC, Cohen SJ, et al. Treating Tobacco Use and Dependence Clinical Practice Guideline. Rockville (MD): US Department of Health and Human Services, Public Health Service; 2000.

Table 2	
Side effects of smoking cessation medications	
Medication	**Side Effects**
Nicotine Gum	Bad taste, throat irritation, mouth sores, hiccups, nausea, jaw discomfort, racing heartbeat, damage to dentures/dental work
Nicotine Lozenge	Trouble sleeping, nausea, hiccups, coughing, heartburn, headache, flatulence (gas)
Nicotine Patch	Skin irritation—redness and itching, dizziness, racing heartbeat, sleep problems or unusual dreams, headache, nausea, vomiting, muscle aches, and stiffness
Nicotine Inhaler	Coughing, throat irritation, upset stomach
Nicotine Nasal Spray	Nasal irritation, runny nose, watery eyes, sneezing, throat irritation, coughing
Bupropion	Changes in appetite, constipation, dizziness, drowsiness, dry mouth, headache, increased sweating, nausea, nervousness, restlessness, taste changes, trouble sleeping, vomiting, weight changes, depressed mood, thoughts of suicide, attempted suicide
Varenicline	Headaches, nausea, vomiting, trouble sleeping, unusual dreams, flatulence (gas), changes in taste, depressed mood, thoughts of suicide, attempted suicide

Adapted from the American Cancer Society Guide to quitting smoking. Available at: http://www. cancer.org/docroot/PED/content/PED_10_13X_Guide_for_Quitting_Smoking.asp. Accessed March 3, 2010.

As previously noted, patches differ in their recommended wear time. Wearing the patch overnight seems to have a clinical advantage in the relief of morning craving but may be more likely to induce sleep disturbances; however, the difference between sleep disturbances related to nocturnal nicotine intake and those related to insufficient nicotine dosing is not always clear. Additionally, in clinical trials, the 24-hour patch yielded greater reductions in anxiety, irritability, and restlessness. Smokers using the 24-hour dosing regimen also experienced longer abstinence than those using the 16-hour patch.[47] For smokers with persistent insomnia and other sleep-related adverse events (particularly vivid dreams), the patches should be removed before bedtime.

The main advantage of nicotine patches is that compliance is simple: the patient simply places the patch on the body in the morning rather than actively using a product throughout the day. For this reason, compliance with patch therapy tends to be higher than for other NRT products.[48] Transdermal patches deliver nicotine more slowly than other NRT formulations, although nicotine plasma concentrations can become higher during the day with patch use.

Importantly, nicotine patches may not adequately protect against acute craving provoked by smoking-related stimuli in all smokers.[49] For people who experience powerful cravings that are not adequately controlled by transdermal nicotine alone, other shorter-acting therapies may be combined to enhance the control of nicotine cravings.

Gum

The first NRT formulation that was made available to consumers was transmucosally delivered nicotine polacrilex (nicotine gum), which has been available since the early 1980s in Europe and 1984 in the United States. The gum is available in 2 doses of

2 mg and 4 mg, delivering approximately 1 mg and 2 mg, respectively.[50] Users are instructed to use a piece of gum every 1 to 2 hours for the first 6 weeks, then to reduce the use to 1 piece every 2 to 4 hours for 3 weeks, and 1 piece every 4 to 8 hours for 3 weeks. Smokers who need an extra piece between doses may use one to respond to episodes of acute craving. Smokers who smoke less than 20 cigarettes per day are instructed to use the 2-mg dose, and those who smoke more are instructed to use the 4-mg dose. In highly dependent smokers, the 4-mg dose is superior to the 2-mg dose.[51] About 50% of nicotine in the gum is absorbed through the buccal mucosa.[50] Thus, when the gum is chewed on a fixed schedule of 10 pieces per day, a smoker receives about 10 or 20 mg of nicotine per day using the 2-or 4-mg gum formulations, respectively. Acidic beverages have been shown to interfere with buccal absorption of nicotine; therefore, patients should avoid consuming acidic beverages (eg, soda, coffee, beer) for 15 minutes before and during chewing gum.

The simple act of chewing a gum is likely to reduce smoking and nicotine cravings.[52] However, after about 15 to 20 minutes of chewing, the nicotine itself reduces craving, and the nicotine gum significantly reduced craving compared with placebo gum. Chewing nicotine gum may cause jaw soreness, which may be reduced by using the "chew and park" method of chewing, whereby the smoker chews the gum to release nicotine and then moves the gum between the cheek and gum for a minute or so. Gum use can also cause a mild burning sensation in the mouth and throat, which some people find undesirable and others find useful in craving relief.

Lozenge

Nicotine lozenges are available in 1- (Europe), 2-, and 4-mg formulations (United States). Unlike nicotine gum in which the smoker chooses the dose based on the number of cigarettes smoked, the indication for the lozenge allocates smokers to the 2- or 4-mg dose based on how soon after waking the first cigarette of the day is smoked. Time to first cigarette is considered a simple but powerful index of nicotine dependence and thus potentially a useful way of determining each smoker's nicotine need.[53]

Like nicotine gum, nicotine from the lozenge is absorbed slowly through the buccal mucosa and delivered into systemic circulation. The lozenge should not be chewed and this is considered a benefit by some patients and a weakness by others who enjoy gum chewing.

Inhaler

The nicotine vapor inhaler is currently marketed as a prescription medication in the United States. The inhaler consists of a mouthpiece and a plastic cartridge containing nicotine. When the inhaler is puffed, nicotine is drawn through the mouthpiece into the mouth of the smoker. The vapor inhaler was designed to satisfy behavioral aspects of smoking, namely, the hand-to-mouth ritual. For some smokers, this may be a useful adjunct. Each inhaler cartridge contains 10 mg nicotine, of which 4 mg is delivered and 2 mg is absorbed. The product is not a true inhaler in that nicotine is not delivered to the bronchi or lungs but deposited and absorbed in the mouth, much like nicotine gum. Nicotine delivery is primarily related to the number of inhalations and ambient temperature, warmer temperatures being more conducive to better nicotine delivery.[54]

Most successful patients in the clinical trials used between 6 and 16 cartridges a day, and the best effect was achieved by frequent bouts of continuous puffing over 20 minutes.[55] The recommended duration of treatment is 3 months, after which patients may be weaned by gradual reduction of the daily dose over the following 6 to

12 weeks. Some patients find the active use requirement too demanding to sustain adequate nicotine levels, whereas for other patients, the frequent puffing and sensory stimuli are an important benefit that helps them manage tobacco cravings.

Nasal Spray

Nicotine nasal spay is marketed as a prescription smoking cessation medication in the United States and in most other countries. The nasal spray was designed to deliver doses of nicotine to the smoker more rapidly than other NRT forms. The device is a multidose bottle with a pump that delivers 0.5 mg of nicotine per squirt. Each dose consists of 2 squirts, 1 to each nostril. Nicotine nasal spray is absorbed into the blood rapidly relative to all other NRT forms.[56]

The dose of nasal spray should be individualized based on the patient's level of nicotine dependence and the occurrence of symptoms of nicotine excess. Patients should be started with 1 or 2 doses per hour, which may be increased up to the maximum of 40 doses per day. Being the NRT form with the most rapid delivery, nasal spray should be able to deliver acute craving relief. The nasal spray may cause some nasal irritation, but this effect dissipates with repeated use in most patients.

Sublingual Tablet

A small nicotine tablet has been developed but is not yet available in the United States. The product is designed to be held under the tongue, where the nicotine in the tablet is absorbed sublingually. The levels of nicotine obtained by use of the 2-mg tablet and 2-mg nicotine gum are similar. It is recommended that smokers use the product for at least 12 weeks, after that the number of tablets used is gradually tapered.

Combination Therapy

One strategy for further improving the efficacy of medications is to combine one medication that allows for passive nicotine delivery (eg, transdermal patch) with another medication that permits acute ad libitum nicotine delivery (eg, gum, nasal spray, inhaler).[57] The rationale for combining NRT medications is that smokers may need both a slow delivery system to achieve a constant concentration of nicotine to relieve cravings and tobacco withdrawal symptoms and a fast-acting preparation to function as rescue medication for immediate relief of breakthrough cravings.[57] Thus, combining the nicotine patch (which may prevent severe withdrawal symptoms) with acute dosing forms (which can provide relief in trigger-to-smoke contexts) may provide an excellent treatment option over either therapy alone.

Bupropion (Zyban) in combination with nicotine patch seems to be more efficacious than nicotine patch alone, possibly because the 2 medications act via different pharmacologic mechanisms.[58] Despite the possibility of increased efficacy, present NRT labeling warns against combination use. Without removal of such warnings, these strategies will be largely limited to smoking cessation specialists and clinics. The complexity of obtaining US FDA approval for combination medications, combined with the difficulty of marketing combination products, has slowed attempts by manufacturers to gain regulatory approval for combination therapies.[57]

Combination therapy need not exclusively include medications. The combination of treatment with bupropion and a customized program of cognitive behavioral therapy (CBT) that is specifically designed to address women's concerns about postcessation weight gain produces higher rates of abstinence at 6 months and longer time to relapse than standard CBT plus bupropion treatment or CBT alone.[59]

Bupropion

Bupropion is a smoking cessation aid that was originally marketed as an antidepressant (Wellbutrin). Its mechanism of action is thought to be related to its effect on norepinephrine and dopamine receptors in the brain.

Clinically, it is possible that bupropion acts by alleviating some of the symptoms of nicotine withdrawal, including depression. Bupropion has been endorsed by the US Clinical Practice Guideline as a first line therapeutic agent.[60] Bupropion has been shown to approximately double the rates of cessation compared with placebo, and the medication is equally effective in men and women.[61] It has also been shown that bupropion combined with nicotine replacement medications may increase cessation rates relative to bupropion alone.[58] The recommended and maximum dose of bupropion is 300 mg/d, given as 150 mg twice daily. Dry mouth and insomnia are the most common adverse events associated with its use. There is a very small risk of seizure, and this risk can be reduced by not prescribing the medication to persons with a history of seizure, with a predisposition toward seizure, or consuming excess alcohol. Bupropion should not be prescribed if any history of serious head injury, bipolar (manic-depressive) illness, or anorexia or bulimia (eating disorders) is present. Serious neuropsychiatric events including, but not limited to, depression, suicidal ideation, suicide attempt, and completed suicide have been reported in patients taking bupropion.[62]

Varenicline

Varenicline (Chantix) is a newer prescription medicine developed to help people stop smoking. It works by interfering with nicotine receptors in the brain and thus has 2 effects: it lessens the pleasurable physical effects a person gets from smoking and it reduces the symptoms of nicotine withdrawal.

Several studies have shown that varenicline can more than double the chances of quitting smoking. Some studies have also found that it may work better than bupropion, at least in the short term.[63,64]

Varenicline is available in pill form and is taken after meals, with a full glass of water. The daily dose increases over the first 8 days of its intake. The dose starts at one 0.5-mg pill a day for the first 3 days, and then the same dose twice a day for the next 4 days. At the start of the second week, the dose is raised to 1 mg each morning and evening. For people who have problems with the higher dose, a lower dose may be used during the quit effort. Varenicline is given for 12 weeks, but people who quit during that time may get another 12 weeks of treatment to boost their chance of staying quit.

Reported side effects of varenicline have included headaches, nausea, vomiting, trouble sleeping, unusual dreams, flatulence (gas), and changes in taste. Serious neuropsychiatric events including, but not limited to, depression, suicidal ideation, suicide attempt, and completed suicide have been reported in patients taking varenicline.[62] People who have these problems should contact their doctors right away. These side effects may happen, but varenicline is usually well tolerated.

Because varenicline is a newer drug, not much research has been done yet to find out if it is safe to use along with NRT products. A recent study has suggested that using varenicline along with NRT is well tolerated and safe.[65]

Other Medications

For those who cannot use any of the US FDA–approved drugs or who have not been able to quit smoking using them, there are other drugs that have shown promise in research studies. They are recommended by the Agency for Healthcare Research and Quality but have not been approved by the US FDA for smoking cessation and are used off-label.[60]

In particular, nortriptyline and clonidine are endorsed by the US Clinical Practice Guideline as agents of second line therapy.[60] Lastly, rimonabant, a drug recently approved to treat obesity in Europe and subsequently withdrawn, has been studied for its potential use in smoking cessation. At present, it is not approved for use in the United States for any indication.[66]

SUMMARY

Nicotine dependence is a significant addiction with many health consequences, causing repercussions throughout the health care industry and beyond. Consistent attempts and efforts at addressing this condition, guiding and advising afflicted patients using motivational techniques and the 5-A stepwise strategies, and instituting appropriate therapies will result in better health outcomes and less incidence of diseases. In pharmacotherapy, NRT and oral medications can be used alone or in combination with varying degrees of success.

REFERENCES

1. Available at: http://www.drugabuse.gov/drugpages/nicotine.html. Accessed March 3, 2010.
2. Available at: http://smoking-quit.info/tobacco-second-major-cause-of-death-worldwide. Accessed March 3, 2010.
3. Centers for Disease Control and Prevention. Annual smoking-attributable mortality, years of potential life lost, and productivity losses—United States, 2000–2004. MMWR Morb Mortal Wkly Rep 2008;57(45):1226–8.
4. Available at: http://www.surgeongeneral.gov/library/secondhandsmoke/. Accessed March 3, 2010.
5. Available at: http://www.cdc.gov/mmwr/preview/mmwrhtml/mm5542a1.htm. Accessed March 3, 2010.
6. Available at: http://pediatrics.aappublications.org/cgi/reprint/124/5/1474. Accessed March 3, 2010.
7. Available at: http://www.cdc.gov/HealthyYouth/tobacco/facts.htm. Accessed March 3, 2010.
8. Available at: http://www.cdc.gov/chronicdisease/resources/publications/fact_sheets/pdf/tobacco.pdf. Accessed March 3, 2010.
9. Available at: http://www.cdc.gov/pcd/issues/2009/jul/08_0153.htm. Accessed March 3, 2010.
10. Lande RGL. Nicotine addiction. e-medicine. March 11, 2010. Available at: http://emedicine.medscape.com/article/287555/. Accessed March 3, 2010.
11. Lasser K, Boyd JW, Woolhandler S, et al. Smoking and mental illness—a population-based prevalence study. JAMA 2000;284:2606–10.
12. Cather C, Barr RS, Evins AE. Smoking and schizophrenia: prevalence, mechanisms and implications for treatment. Clin Schizophr Relat Psychoses 2008;2(1):70–8.
13. Evins AE. Nicotine dependence in schizophrenia: prevalence, mechanisms, and implications for treatment. Psychiatr Times 25(3):1–2.
14. Corvin A, O'Mahoney E, O'Regan M, et al. Cigarette smoking and psychotic symptoms in bipolar affective disorder. Br J Psychiatry 2001;179:35–8.
15. Available at: http://www.cdc.gov/tobacco/data_statistics/sgr/2004/pdfs/executive summary.pdf. Accessed March 3, 2010.

16. Available at: http://www.cancer.org/docroot/AA/content/AA_2_5_5x_Global_Tobacco_Epidemic.asp. Accessed March 3, 2010.
17. Richter P, Pechacek T, Swahn M, et al. Reducing levels of toxic chemicals in cigarette smoke: a new healthy people 2010 objective. Public Health Rep 2008;123(1):30–8.
18. Available at: http://www.epa.gov/smokefree/pubs/etsfs.html. Accessed March 3, 2010.
19. Lee JH. Smokeless tobacco and head and neck cancer: there is risk even without fire. S D Med 2009;(Spec No):38–9.
20. Available at: http://www.cancer.org/docroot/ped/content/ped_10_2x_secondhand_smoke-clean_indoor_air.asp. Accessed March 3, 2010.
21. Available at: http://health.nytimes.com/health/guides/disease/chronic-obstructive-pulmonary-disease/print.html. Accessed March 3, 2010.
22. Cropp AJ. COPD and emphysema. In: Domino FJ, editor. The 5-minute clinical consult. 17th edition. Philadelphia (PA): Lippincott Williams & Wilkins; 2009. p. 280–1.
23. Tiemstra J. Chronic obstructive pulmonary disease. FP Essentials, Edition No. 355, AAFP Home Study. Leawood (KS): American Academy of Family Physicians; 2008. p. 24.
24. Available at: http://cme.medscape.com/viewarticle/578143. Accessed March 3, 2010.
25. Available at: http://www.americanheart.org/presenter.jhtml?identifier=4545. Accessed March 3, 2010.
26. Available at: http://www.who.int/tobacco/en/atlas8.pdf. Accessed March 3, 2010.
27. Gu D, Kelly TN, Wu X. Mortality attributable to smoking in China. N Engl J Med 2009;360(2):150–9.
28. Available at: http://www.medscape.com/viewarticle/717666. Accessed March 3, 2010.
29. Rehan VK, Asotra K, Torday JS. The effects of smoking on the developing lung: insights from a biologic model for lung development, homeostasis, and repair. Lung 2009;187(5):281–9.
30. Anderson ME, Johnson DC, Batal HA. Sudden infant death syndrome and prenatal maternal smoking: rising attributed risk in the back to sleep era. BMC Med 2005;3:4.
31. Preshaw PM, Heasman L, Stacey F, et al. The effect of quitting smoking on chronic periodontitis. J Clin Periodontol 2005;32:869–79.
32. Available at: http://www.cascadeeyemds.com/docs/diseases/SmokingandEye Disease.pdf. Accessed March 3, 2010.
33. Available at: http://www.simplyantiaging.com/820/smoking-and-skin-aging/. Accessed March 3, 2010.
34. Gades NM, Nehra A, Jacobson DJ, et al. Association between smoking and erectile dysfunction: a population-based study. Am J Epidemiol 2005;161:346–51.
35. Wilks DJ, Hay AWM. Smoking and female fecundity: the effect and importance of study design. Eur J Obstet Gynecol Reprod Biol 2004;112:127–35.
36. Pasqualotto FF, Lucon AM, Sobreiro BP, et al. Effects of medical therapy, alcohol, smoking, and endocrine disruptors on male infertility. Rev Hosp Clin Fac Med Sao Paulo 2004;59(6):375–82.
37. U.S. Preventive Services Task Force. Counseling and interventions to prevent tobacco use and tobacco-caused disease in adults and pregnant women: U.S. Preventive Services Task Force reaffirmation recommendation statement. Ann Intern Med 2009;150(8):551–5.

38. Quinn VP, Hollis JF, Smith KS, et al. Effectiveness of the 5-As tobacco cessation treatments in nine HMOs. J Gen Intern Med 2009;24(2):149–54.
39. Lai DT, Cahill K, Qin Y, et al. Motivational interviewing for smoking cessation. Cochrane Database Syst Rev 2010;1:CD006936.
40. Henningfield JE, Fant RV, Buchhalter AR, et al. Pharmacotherapy for nicotine dependence. CA Cancer J Clin 2005;55:281–99.
41. Molyneux A. Nicotine replacement therapy. BMJ 2004;328(7437):454–6.
42. Rose JE. Nicotine and non-nicotine factors in cigarette addiction. Psychopharmacology 2006;184:274–85.
43. Rose JE, Behm FM, Westman EC, et al. Pharmacologic and sensorimotor components of satiation in cigarette smoking. Pharmacol Biochem Behav 2003;76:243–50.
44. Brauer LH, Behm FM, Lane JD, et al. Individual differences in smoking reward from denicotinized cigarettes. Nicotine Tob Res 2001;3:101–9.
45. Stead LF, Perera R, Bullen C, et al. Nicotine replacement therapy for smoking cessation. Cochrane Database Syst Rev 2008;1:CD000146.
46. Kozlowski LT, Giovino GA, Edwards B, et al. Advice on using over-the-counter nicotine replacement therapy-patch, gum, or lozenge-to quit smoking. Addict Behav 2007;32(10):2140–50.
47. Shiffman S, Elash CA, Paton SM, et al. Comparative efficacy of 24-hour and 16-hour transdermal nicotine patches for relief of morning craving. Addiction 2000;95(8):1185–95.
48. Hajek P, West R, Foulds J, et al. Randomized comparative trial of nicotine polacrilex, a transdermal patch, nasal spray, and an inhaler. Arch Intern Med 1999;159:2033–8.
49. Tiffany ST, Cox LS, Elash CA. Effects of transdermal nicotine patches on abstinence-induced and cue-elicited craving in cigarette smokers. J Consult Clin Psychol 2000;68:233–40.
50. Benowitz NL, Jacob P III, Savanapridi C. Determinants of nicotine intake while chewing nicotine polacrilex gum. Clin Pharmacol Ther 1987;41:467–73.
51. Herrera N, Franco R, Herrera L, et al. Nicotine gum, 2 and 4 mg, for nicotine dependence. A double-blind placebo-controlled trial within a behavior modification support program. Chest 1995;108:447–51.
52. Cohen LM, Collins FL, Britt DM. The effect of chewing gum on tobacco withdrawal. Addict Behav 1997;22:769–73.
53. Heatherton TF, Kozlowski LT, Frecker RC, et al. The Fagerström test for nicotine dependence: a revision of the Fagerström tolerance questionnaire. Br J Addict 1991;86:1119–27.
54. Lunell E, Molander L, Andersson SB. Temperature dependency of the release and bioavailability of nicotine from a nicotine vapour inhaler; in vitro/in vivo correlation. Eur J Clin Pharmacol 1997;52:495–500.
55. Bolliger CT, Zellweger JP, Danielsson T, et al. Smoking reduction with oral nicotine inhalers: double blind, randomised clinical trial of efficacy and safety. BMJ 2000;321:329–33.
56. Schneider NG, Lunell E, Olmstead RE, et al. Clinical pharmacokinetics of nasal nicotine delivery. A review and comparison to other nicotine systems. Clin Pharmacokinet 1996;31:65–80.
57. Sweeney CT, Fant RV, Fagerstrom KO, et al. Combination nicotine replacement therapy for smoking cessation: rationale, efficacy and tolerability. CNS Drugs 2001;15:453–67.

58. Jorenby DE, Leischow SJ, Nides MA, et al. A controlled trial of sustained-release bupropion, a nicotine patch, or both for smoking cessation. N Engl J Med 1999; 340:685–91.
59. Available at: http://www.medscape.com/viewarticle/719288. Accessed March 3, 2010.
60. Fiore MC, Jaen CR, Baker TB, et al. Treating tobacco use and dependence: 2008 update. Rockville (MD): U.S. Department of Health and Human Services, Public Health Service; 2008. p. 257.
61. Scharf D, Shiffman S. Are there gender differences in smoking cessation, with and without bupropion? Pooled- and meta-analyses of clinical trials of Bupropion SR. Addiction 2004;99:1462–9.
62. Physicians Desk Reference, 2010. Montvale (NJ): PDR Network; 2010. p. 1762, 2712.
63. Hays JT, Ebbert JO, Sood A. Efficacy and safety of varenicline for smoking cessation. Am J Med 2008;121(4 Suppl 1):S32–42.
64. Nides M, Glover FD, Reus VI, et al. Varenicline versus bupropion SR or placebo for smoking cessation: a pooled analysis. Am J Health Behav 2008; 32:664–75.
65. Ebbert JO, Burke MV, Hays JT. Combination treatment with varenicline and nicotine replacement therapy. Nicotine Tob Res 2009;11(5):572–6.
66. Cahill K, Ussher MH. Cannabinoid type 1 receptor antagonists (rimonabant) for smoking cessation. Cochrane Database Syst Rev 2007;4:CD005353.

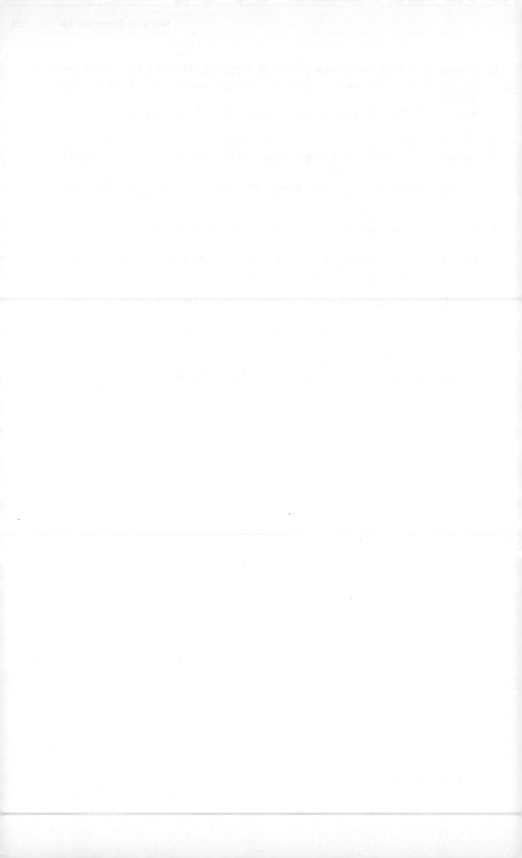

Stimulant Abuse: Pharmacology, Cocaine, Methamphetamine, Treatment, Attempts at Pharmacotherapy

Daniel Ciccarone, MD, MPH

KEYWORDS

• Stimulants • Cocaine • Amphetamine • Methamphetamine

STIMULANT USE AND ABUSE: A PRIMARY CARE ISSUE
Recent History

Stimulants, including cocaine and amphetamines, are among the most widely used and abused illegal substances in the United States. Coca chewing has a long history of indigenous use in South America.[1] Widespread use of cocaine followed its isolation from coca in 1859 and a medical publication purporting its benefits in 1884. The subsequent incorporation of cocaine into patent medicines and popular beverages, for example, Vin Mariani and Coca-Cola, contributed to its profligate use.[2] Rising social and medical problems raised concern in many circles, and restrictions were gradually applied until the Harrison Act (1914) banned all over-the-counter (OTC) inclusion of cocaine.[3] In the United States, a popularity wave of cocaine use began in the 1970s followed by the crack wave of the 1980s.[4] These waves have left paths of adverse consequences, including association with the human immunodeficiency virus (HIV) epidemic, in the latter decades of the twentieth century.

The first of the synthetic stimulants, amphetamine (isolated in 1887), was first popularized in the 1930s with an OTC nasal decongestant (ie, Benzedrine inhaler) containing the amphetamine phenylisopropylamine and the following discoveries of clinical applications for fatigue, narcolepsy, and depression.[5] High availability and popularity led to misuse, and OTC use was banned in 1957. Prescription misuse followed World War II (with common military usage) and illicit diversion of medications. Methamphetamine (isolated in 1919) use peaked during the late 1960s, creating a "speed scene."

This work was supported by Grant DA16165, from the National Institutes of Health, National Institute on Drug Abuse.
Department of Family and Community Medicine, University of California San Francisco, 500 Parnassus Avenue, MU-3E, Box 0900, San Francisco, CA 94143-0900, USA
E-mail address: ciccaron@fcm.ucsf.edu

Prim Care Clin Office Pract 38 (2011) 41–58
doi:10.1016/j.pop.2010.11.004   **primarycare.theclinics.com**

The passage of the Controlled Substances Act in 1971 led to a dramatic decline in prescribed amphetamine, and the popularity of amphetamines and methamphetamine declined for a time.[6] The 1990s brought a reemergence of methamphetamine, particularly to the western United States, concurrent to mounting small scale production, aka "meth labs," first in California and subsequently spreading nationwide.[7] New forms of methamphetamine, for example, "crank" and "ice," have had their popularity waves as well. The popularity of amphetamines is reciprocal with cultural representations throughout the 1940s to 1990s, for example, in literature, movies, and music.[8,9]

Epidemiology

According to the 2008 National Survey on Drug Use and Health (NSDUH), the national prevalence of current cocaine use is third after marijuana and misuse of prescription medications. The estimated lifetime prevalence of cocaine use is 14.7% in the US population 12 years or older (3.4%, crack use prevalence). Current use (past month) of cocaine was reported by 0.7% of persons 12 years and older in 2008, decreasing significantly from 1.0% in 2003. The proportion reporting current crack use, 0.1%, also decreased from the levels in 2003 (0.3%).[10] The NSDUH may underreport drug use in certain populations, including the homeless, institutionalized persons, and college students.

According to the 2008 NSDUH, the estimated lifetime prevalence of nonmedical amphetamine use is 8.5% in the US population, down from 9.7% in 2003. Current use of all amphetamines is reported at 0.4% (2008), down from 0.6% (2003); only 0.1% of the population reports current methamphetamine use in the latest survey, which has decreased from 0.3%. Methamphetamine use is more prevalent in the western United States but is trending eastward.[11]

The Drug Abuse Warning Network (DAWN) is a national survey of nonfederal short-stay hospitals with 24-hour emergency departments (EDs) of patient visits associated with drug misuse or abuse; DAWN has a separate survey of medical examiner data on mortality related to illegal drug use. According to the 2006 DAWN survey, 1 in 3 (31%) of all drug-related emergency visits involved cocaine; methamphetamine was associated with 5% of all drug-related ED visits and amphetamine, 2%. No statistically significant change in stimulant-related ED mentions was noted over the past 2 annual surveys.[12] In the DAWN mortality state profiles, cocaine was 1 of the top 3 drugs involved in drug-related deaths in 6 of 10 states; stimulants (amphetamines and methamphetamine) ranked in the top 10, of mortality-involved drugs, in 6 of 10 states, with 4 being western states.[13] Although household surveys report low methamphetamine use prevalence, regional law enforcement agencies are reporting heightened concerns. In addition, the associated economic and societal costs of methamphetamine use are estimated to be high.[14]

FORMS, PREPARATION, AND USE
Cocaine

Cocaine is a naturally occurring alkaloid in the leaves of the coca plant, *Erythroxylon coca*, which is indigenous to the Andean region of South America. The area of coca under cultivation in Colombia, Peru and Bolivia peaked in 2000 at 221,300 hectares, subsequently declining to 167,600 hectares in 2008. Most of the cocaine derived from this harvest is for export. Estimates of potential cocaine production for the region have varied little since 1994; in that year, the estimated production was 891 metric tons. Since peaking in 2000 at 1008 metric tons, there has been a decline to 845 metric tons in 2008. Global cocaine seizures have risen dramatically in the last decade; in 2007, about 711 metric tons of street-level cocaine was seized, double the amount in 2000. Adjusting for purity, an estimated 42% of global pure cocaine was reportedly confiscated in 2007.[15]

Cocaine is street-available in both acidic (salt) and basic forms.[16] Cocaine hydrochloride (aka "coke," "blow," "snow," "nose candy," "yayo")[17] is a water-soluble powder with a high melting point. As such, it is bioavailable (approximately 30%–60%) through insufflation (ie, snorting or "tooting") or easily dissolved for intravenous injection; it is not usually smoked because the active ingredient is destroyed by the temperatures required for vaporization. Time to peak subjective effect averages 14.6 minutes after insufflation compared with 3.1 minutes after injection.[18] Nasal absorption is limited because of the vasoconstrictive properties of cocaine.

Base cocaine, aka "crack," or "rock,"[17] can be vaporized and inhaled owing to its lower melting point. The term crack reportedly comes from the sound the material makes while melting.[6] Since its entry into the US market in 1985, crack cocaine spread rapidly because of its low cost and rapid action. The time to reach peak subjective effect is significantly faster for smoked cocaine (1.4 min) than for intravenous or insufflated cocaine.[18] In the 1980s street doses were frequently seen in US cities, selling for as little as $2.50 to $5.00.[19] Crack cocaine largely replaced an outmoded base form called "freebase," which involved a complicated series of dangerous steps to solubilize and extract base cocaine from its hydrochloride salt.

The average purity of cocaine available on the US streets was approximately 60% in 2007.[20] Diluents, that is, fillers or "cut," include simple sugars, for example, dextrose, starch, or white inert powders, such as, talc. Adulterants, which may have some additive or mimicking active effects, include topical anesthetics, such as procaine, and cheaper stimulants, such as caffeine or ephedrine.[21] Reports of adverse consequences from cocaine tainted with levamisole (a veterinary medication) have risen recently.[22,23] Cocaine is frequently used by heroin-dependent users in combination, aka "speedball." Tobacco, alcohol, and marijuana are frequently used in conjunction with cocaine.

Amphetamine-Methamphetamine

Historically, US illicit methamphetamine came from small producers in Mexico and California. The 1990s saw growth and spread in the domestic production of methamphetamine. Domestic methamphetamine seizures by the Drug Enforcement Administration increased dramatically from 272 kg in 1990 to 1549 kg in 2008 after peaking at 2161 kg in 2005.[24] The number of US methamphetamine laboratory seizures increased from 7025 in 2000 to 10249 in 2003, declining to 2584 in 2008.[20] Much of this decline has been offset by increased importation of methamphetamine from Mexico. Methamphetamine can be made from OTC nasal decongestant products containing ephedrine and pseudoephedrine. For this reason, strict controls have been placed on OTC purchases as well as other precursor supplies. Since 2004, 44 states have restricted sales.[25] Since 2005, the government of Mexico has progressively increased precursor controls with some measurable effect on production.[20]

Methamphetamine exists in 2 stereoisomer, that is, L and D, forms. L-Methamphetamine has peripheral α-adrenergic activity and has been used in the past as a nasal decongestant (ie, Vicks inhaler). D-Methamphetamine (aka "speed," "crystal," "meth," or "crank") is a powerful stimulant with 3 to 5 times the central nervous system (CNS) activity as the L-isomer and a half-life of 10 to 12 hours (cocaine's half-life is 0.5–2.0 hours).[26] The D isomer can be insufflated, smoked, injected, or inserted per rectum. Its forms are powder (usually white, but may be of other colors) or crystalline.

Ice (aka "glass," or "Tina") is a highly purified form of D-methamphetamine, which is intended for smoking; it vaporizes at an even lower temperature than crack cocaine.[27,28]

Amphetamines-Other

Several synthetic stimulants, including amphetamine and methylphenidate, are available as prescription drugs. Forms include tablets, capsules, liquids, and patches. Indications include attention-deficit/hyperactivity disorder (ADHD), weight control, and narcolepsy. OTC stimulants include aerosolized or ingested forms of decongestants as well as caffeine in multifarious forms.[29] There has been a recent boom of highly caffeinated beverages, aka "energy" drinks.[30]

Diversion of prescription stimulants is a concern. Given the increase in the diagnosis of ADHD, the number of prescriptions for stimulant medication has grown. Surveys of college students reveal that the illicit use of stimulants has grown recently and this use is at its highest level in decades.[31] However, there is no evidence that appropriate medical use of prescription stimulant medication leads to increased drug abuse. Although studies examining cohorts of persons with ADHD confirm high prevalences of adult comorbid substance use disorders, they also find that treatment with stimulant medication is not associated with increased substance abuse in adulthood.[32]

OTC stimulant-based appetitive suppressants have also raised concern over the past 2 decades. Fenfluramine-phentermine (aka fen-phen) was a combination stimulant medication widely advertised and popular in the 1990s. The adverse association of this medication with cardiac valvular regurgitation and pulmonary hypertension led to its removal from the market in 1997.[33] An OTC decongestant and appetite suppressant, phenylpropanolamine, was removed from the market in 2005 after its association with hemorrhagic stroke among women was found.[34]

EFFECTS ON NEUROTRANSMITTER SYSTEMS

Stimulants facilitate the activity of the monoamine neurotransmitters, that is, dopamine, norepinephrine, and serotonin, in the CNS and peripheral nervous system.[35,36] Both cocaine and amphetamines act on presynaptic monoamine reuptake transporters but each in unique ways. Cocaine is a reuptake inhibitor, that is, it blocks the action of the reuptake transporter, thus allowing more neurotransmitters to stay active in the synapse. Amphetamines are releasers, that is, they are taken up by the transporter in exchange for neurotransmitter release into the synapse.

The reward circuit of the CNS includes dopamine pathways extending from the ventral tegmental area of the midbrain to the prefrontal cortex and limbic regions, including the shell of the nucleus accumbens and ventral pallidum, with the key areas for stimulant reward being the prefrontal cortex and nucleus accumbens. Animal and human studies support the role of dopaminergic activity, particularly in these pathways, as mediating the behavioral effects of stimulants.[36] Cocaine and amphetamine intakes transiently increase extracellular dopamine concentrations in the reward circuit.[37] Affinity for the dopamine transporter is correlated to behavioral reinforcing effects in animal studies of varying stimulant potencies.[38] Genetically engineered mice with dopamine transporters altered to not bind cocaine show no reinforcing effects of cocaine administration.[39] Likewise, knockout mice lacking dopamine D_1 receptors do not self-administer cocaine.[40] In human positron emission tomographic studies, increases in dorsal striatum dopamine are associated with self-reported euphoric responses to short-term stimulant use as well as to conditioned drug cues.[37] Blockade of more than half the dopamine transporters is required to reduce the psychological or behavioral effects of stimulants.[41] Thus, studies of dopamine receptor antagonists (eg, antipsychotic medications) or synthesis inhibitors usually fail because of intolerance to the experimental drugs' effects.[42]

Stimulants also increase serotonin and norepinephrine activity and have effects on several other neurotransmitter systems. Serotonin enhancement is contributory, but not obligatory, in the behavioral rewarding from stimulant use.[43] The subjective effects of stimulants of varying potencies are correlated with norepinephrine release.[44] Glutamate may play an important role in relapse to cocaine or amphetamine abuse.[45] Environmental cues and drug seeking leading to glutamatergic upregulation is a proposed model. Stimulants also increase acetylcholine release in the brain and may play a role in reward pathways.[46]

CLINICAL FEATURES
Short-Term Use: Intoxication and Overdose

The clinical effects of stimulant use, including psychological, behavioral and physiologic effects, vary by short-term versus long-term use, potency of drug, route of administration, and dosage.

Short-term use of stimulants leads to rapid neurotransmitter release, resulting in euphoria, increased energy and libido, reduced fatigue and appetite, and behavioral responses, for example, increased self-confidence and alertness.[47] Acute adrenergic effects include dose-responsive tachycardia and elevated blood pressure. Dose-equivalent responses to cocaine are seen with approximately 15 to 25 mg injected intravenously or smoked, 40 to 100 mg insufflated, or 100 to 200 mg ingested; oral amphetamine is approximately 10 times more potent per milligram.[48]

With escalating effective dose (ie, by greater potency or amount or more efficient route), there is greater euphoria at first but also increased likelihood of toxic and dysphoric effects, including insomnia, anxiety, irritability, confusion, paranoia, panic attacks, and hallucinations; related behavioral consequences include impulsivity and grandiosity.[49,50] Acute adrenergic side-effects include hyperpyrexia, hyperreflexia, tremor, diaphoresis, tachycardia, hypertension, and tachypnea.[51] Overdose may manifest in convulsions, cerebral hemorrhage or infarct, cardiac arrhythmias or ischemia, respiratory failure, and muscle overactivity leading to rhabdomyolysis.[52]

Long-Term Use

Long-term use of stimulants is frequently performed in binge-abstinence cycles. Cycles of use can last 12 or so hours (typically cocaine) to several days (methamphetamine). This finding is reported in epidemiologic studies[53,54] as well as animal studies.[55]

Cyclical use, drug craving, and relapse may be explained by the concept of sensitization,[56] which occurs when intermittent use of a drug leads to enhanced effects. Because the enhanced effects are often desired, cyclical use is learned and practiced. Repeated phasic use of low-dose cocaine may lead to increased sensitivity, including startle reactions, repetitive and stereotyped behaviors, and alteration of motor function.[57] There is cross-sensitization among stimulants in that prior amphetamine administration subsequently boosts the effects of cocaine.[58]

Some of the most prominent and disturbing effects of escalating stimulant use include a spectrum of psychotic features, including paranoia, delusions, and hallucinations.[59] Hallucinations include tactile hallucinations or formication, colloquially referred to as "tweaking," in which users commonly pick at their skin or perform other repetitive searching behaviors.[60] About 25% to 50% of long-term stimulant users report experiencing psychotic symptoms, and sensitization may worsen these with continued use.[49,61,62] Psychotic symptoms may also persist for years after abstinence from amphetamine use,[63] with flashbacks reported by methamphetamine users up to 2 years after last use.[64]

In time, neurotransmitter down-regulation can occur, leading to an array of clinical features. Tolerance to the psychological and physical effects of stimulants may develop after several doses or within weeks.[48,65] Imaging studies reveal decreased dopamine release and receptor availability in long-term users.[37] Changes in brain structure, for example, decreased frontal cortex volume and enlarged basal ganglia, are also associated with long-term cocaine use.[66] Cognitive impairment may result and persist for months after abstinence.[67]

Withdrawal from cocaine and amphetamine produces such a strong backlash of psychological and behavioral symptoms that it is frequently referred to as a "crash." Acute withdrawal symptoms include hypersomnolence, strong cravings, and depression. These symptoms may be followed by a several week period of dysphoria, lethargy, and anhedonia.[68,69] Relapses are common owing to environmental cueing and the stark contrast between "high" and "crash" states.

Addiction

The potential for misuse, dependence, and abuse of stimulants is high. Surveys of persons not in treatment estimate that 10% to 15% of stimulant users become dependent[70]; in treatment-seeking populations, the proportion exceeds 50%.[71] Heavier use is clearly related to dependency, but route of use is also a key factor; stimulant smokers and injectors are more likely to become dependent.[72] Faster pharmacokinetics (eg, smoked over ingested routes) and shorter peak to trough cycles (eg, cocaine over methamphetamine) aid abuse potential.[73]

The American Psychiatric Association's *Diagnostic and Statistical Manual of Mental Disorder, Fourth Edition, Text Revision* requires that several criteria be met for the diagnosis of stimulant abuse. The criteria include evidence of a maladaptive pattern of use, clinically significant impairment, and more than one of the following (in a 12-month period): (1) failure to fulfill major role obligations, (2) use in physically hazardous situations, (3) recurrent legal problems, and (4) continued use despite social and interpersonal problems.[74]

The variability seen in individuals' responses to stimulants may be because of genetics, personality traits, or social/environmental cues (eg, drug use setting) as well as a variety of other factors. The role of genetics is supported by twin studies in which identical twins are highly concordant in the response to short-term stimulant intake, in the initiation of stimulants, and in stimulant dependence and abuse.[75]

Medical Complications

The medical consequences of stimulant abuse are many and occur in all major organ systems (**Table 1**). One way of understanding and categorizing these problems is by mechanism of injury, for example, ischemia, nervous system stimulation, direct toxicity and so forth.

Mechanisms leading to tissue ischemia include vasoconstriction, vasospasm, endothelial damage, and clotting stimulation (eg, increased platelet activation and aggregation).[76] Stimulant use is associated with cerebrovascular disease and injury, including hemorrhagic and ischemic strokes[51]; myocardial infarction (all aforementioned reasons plus increased oxygen demand)[77]; renal failure (secondary to ischemia or rhabdomyolysis)[78]; gastrointestinal disease (eg, ulceration and intestinal infarction)[76,79]; muscle damage (also possible direct toxicity, leading to

Table 1
Medical complications of stimulant use

Organ System/Organ	Acute Complications	Chronic Complications
CNS	Hallucinations, especially tactile; dyskinesia; seizures	Psychotic symptoms; cerebrovascular disease/stroke; movement disorders, eg, dystonic reactions, akathisia, choreoathetosis, tardive dyskinesia
Cardiovascular System	Tachycardia, hypertension, myocardial infarction, arrhythmias	Myocarditis, cardiomyopathy, myocardial fibrosis, myocardial infarction
Pulmonary System	Cough, shortness of breath, wheezing, pulmonary edema, hemorrhage, pneumothorax	Interstitial pneumonitis, bronchiolitis obliterans
Renal System	—	Renal ischemia, renal failure
Gastrointestinal System	Reduced gastric motility	Gastric ulceration and perforation, intestinal infarction, ischemic colitis
Liver	—	Viral hepatitis secondary to contaminated syringe use
Endocrine System	Reduced prolactin; increased epinephrine, CRH, ACTH, cortisol, and LH	Increased, normal, or decreased prolactin; normal testosterone, cortisol, LH, and thyroid hormones
Musculoskeletal System	Movement disorders (see CNS)	Rhabdomyolysis
Head and Neck	Rhinitis	Rhinitis, perforated nasal septum, nasal and gingival ulceration, sinusitis, dental decay and periodontal disease, xerostomia, corneal ulcers
Immune System	—	Vasculitis syndromes
Sexual Function	—	Erectile dysfunction, irregular menses
Reproductive System	Vaginal bleeding, abruption placenta, premature rupture of membranes	FDA category C, placenta previa, low birth weight
General/Other	Dehydration	Weight loss, nutritional deficits

Abbreviations: ACTH, adrenocorticotropic hormone; CRH, corticotropin-releasing hormone; FDA, Food and Drug Administration; LH, luteinizing hormone.

rhabdomyolysis, with up to one-third of patients developing acute renal failure)[76,80]; nasal and sinus damages[81]; and reproductive complications (eg, abruption placenta, low birth weight, and feeding difficulties; concerns persist regarding infant cognitive deficits but longer-term studies are somewhat reassuring).[82–84]

Excess nervous system stimulation secondary to stimulant use is associated with seizures (usually tonic-clonic),[76,85] movement disorders (increased basal ganglia dopaminergic activity resulting in repetitive behaviors [aka tweaking], acute dystonic reactions, dyskinesia, and akathisia),[48,86] and psychotic symptoms[63,87] (both through dopaminergic excess[88] and focal perfusion deficits [methamphetamine][89]). Sympathetic nervous system stimulation leads to tachycardia and elevated blood pressure,[51] endocrine stimulation or inhibition (eg, dopamine inhibition of pituitary prolactin),[90] and sexual dysfunction.[91]

Stimulant use may cause direct tissue toxicities resulting in associations with cardiac arrhythmias (secondary to sodium channel blockade and increased norepinephrine),[92,93] myocarditis and cardiomyopathy (toxic effect of drug or from long-term exposure to high levels of catecholamines),[92,94] and pulmonary symptoms and disease (from acute shortness of breath to pulmonary edema, presumably because of combination of direct toxicity and vascular changes).[95,96]

The pathophysiology of many of these adverse organ events is incompletely understood, and many have overlapping causes. In addition, some may be because of, or exacerbated by, drug contamination or may be secondary to lifestyle (eg, malnutrition) and social/environmental factors. A good example is "meth mouth," dental and periodontal decay caused by a combination of tissue shrinkage, poor fluid and high sugar intakes, and neglect.[97]

HIV

Use of stimulants is associated with HIV infection through drug and sexual risk takings as well as though social mechanisms, such as poverty and sexual power dynamics. Drug injection is a well-known risk, with transmission increased by syringe/needle and paraphernalia sharing.[98] Cocaine use is associated with increased frequency of injection and needle sharing.[99] Injection risk behaviors also increase transmission risk for other viruses, including hepatitis C virus and hepatitis B virus; hepatitis C virus has a particularly high incidence among injection drug users.[100]

Sexual risk (including risk taking and imposed social/power risk) is also increased among cocaine users, with reported increased numbers of partners, increased frequency of unprotected intercourse, and exchange of sex for money or drugs.[101] Use of crack cocaine was independently associated with HIV infection in a large epidemiologic study; transmission is likely through the confluence of poverty and sexual risk.[102]

Use of methamphetamine is also associated with sexual risk taking leading to HIV infection and other sexually transmitted diseases (STDs) in both heterosexual and men-who-have-sex-with-men (MSM) populations.[103] Urban MSM have a much higher prevalence of methamphetamine use than that in the general population.[104] In MSM cohort studies, methamphetamine use is associated with unprotected anal intercourse.[105,106] In a cross-sectional study of MSM, methamphetamine use concurrent with unprotected anal intercourse was an independent risk factor for recent HIV seroconversion.[107] The use of erectile dysfunction medications, such as sildenafil citrate (Viagra), in the "party and play" scene is creating concern.[103] The combination of erectile dysfunction medication (or amyl/butyl nitrate, aka "poppers") and methamphetamine is considered a sexual performance duo; the erectile dysfunction drug counters one of the common consequences of methamphetamine use.[108] This combination unfortunately leads to increased sexual risk taking,[109] STDs,[110] and HIV seroconversion.[111]

TREATMENT
Screening

In the primary care setting, substance use concerns lie in a continuum of risk, and many patients with low to moderate substance use disorders present subclinically. Screening for at-risk levels of alcohol use in the primary care setting has been given a B rating (recommended based on fair evidence) by the United States Preventive Services Task Force (USPSTF).[112] However, according to the USPSTF, the benefit and clinical utility of screening asymptomatic patients for illicit substance use remains unclear.[113] Other professional groups, for example, the American Academy of Pediatrics, recommend identification of adolescents at risk for substance use disorders,[114] and the American College of Obstetrics and Gynecology recommends screening of pregnant women.[115] Many validated screening instruments exist, such as CAGE-AID (cut down, annoyed, guilty, eye opener adapted to include drugs), AUDIT (Alcohol Use Disorders Identification Test; including adaptations for illicit drug screening), and DAST (Drug Abuse Screening Test). Given the time and resource constraints, a consensus panel has recommended a single screening question, "Have you used street drugs more than five times in your life?"[116] Another single screening question has been recently tested for use in primary care settings (Dr R. Saitz), "How many times in the past year have you used an illegal drug or used a prescription medication for non-medical reasons?"[117]

Screening, brief interventions, and referral to treatment (SBIRT) is a clinical model with a growing evidence base. Brief intervention, focusing on risk reduction, involves client-centered counseling sessions assessing motivation to change, reflection on the personal consequences of drug use, and setting of treatment goals. The FRAMES (Feedback, Responsibility, Advice, Menu of treatment options, Empathic and Self-Efficacy) model using motivational interviewing is a key technique.[118] The evidence for the effectiveness of screening and brief interventions is extensive for reducing risky alcohol use[119–121] and is evolving for addressing substance misuse. An evaluation of a large multisite federally funded SBIRT service program found significant reductions in the proportion of patients using illicit drugs, including cocaine and methamphetamine, at 6-months follow-up.[122] Additional studies support brief motivational intervention in reducing cocaine[123] and amphetamine use.[124] The adoption of 2008 Medicare and Medicaid billing codes should facilitate dissemination of SBIRT in primary care settings.[117]

Behavioral/Social

Behavioral and psychosocial approaches are the mainstays of treatment of stimulant dependence, whereas pharmacologic treatment remains elusive (see the following section).[125] These approaches include cognitive behavioral therapy, community reinforcement approach, contingency management, as well as combinations of these and other approaches. A meta-analysis of psychosocial treatments for cocaine abuse found a statistically borderline, but moderate, reduction in combined dependency outcomes.[126] Cognitive behavioral therapy focuses on learning strategies to change maladaptive patterns and increase coping skills; relapse prevention is a common goal. For cocaine dependence, use of cognitive behavioral therapy has been shown to be more effective than less intensive approaches,[127–129] particularly for those with greater disease burden.[130] A recent review showed the effectiveness of cognitive behavioral therapy for the treatment of methamphetamine dependence.[131]

Contingency management is one of the most promising approaches for the treatment of substance use disorders, including cocaine and methamphetamine abuse. The conceptual foundation of contingency management is based in operant conditioning, the study of how systematically applied conditions affect voluntary behavior. Artificially applied conditions are designed to either reinforce or punish a set of defined behaviors (eg, drug use) to achieve a defined behavioral goal (eg, drug abstinence).[132]

Contingency management falls on a spectrum of behavioral treatment options available in substance use treatment. Contingency management is unique in that it uses contrived reinforcements to achieve the explicit goal of short-term drug abstinence. These reinforcements commonly include financial reward or the use of vouchers for goods and services, for example, housing. This management differs from a community reinforcement approach, which focuses on natural social reinforcements that exist in the community, for example, support from a social group or praise from a spouse.

The effectiveness of contingency management for substance use treatment is supported by several meta-analyses.[126,133–135] For the treatment of cocaine dependence, effectiveness of contingency management has been shown in a meta-analysis[134] and several randomized control trials.[136–138] Combining contingency management with cognitive behavioral therapy revealed no clear benefit from contingency management alone.[136] A community reinforcement approach combined with vouchers looks promising.[139] One persistent concern is that the effects of contingency management are short-lived, that is, the benefits diminish once the vouchers are removed. In a study of contingency management versus cognitive behavioral therapy for stimulant dependence, contingency management was superior during the trial phase but cognitive behavioral therapy was equivalent in effect once the trial was over.[140] Contingency management combined with cognitive behavioral therapy improved abstinence among methamphetamine users.[141] In a population of gay and bisexual men, contingency management improved methamphetamine use risk, whereas a culturally modified cognitive behavioral approach reduced sexual risk behavior.[142] A review of behavioral and psychosocial treatments for stimulant use found no evidence for difference in treatment efficacy between the management of cocaine and methamphetamine use.[125]

Pharmacologic

At present, no medication is approved by the US Food and Drug Administration for use in cocaine or amphetamine dependence. Numerous classes of medication have been studied, primarily in small clinical trials. Antidepressants, including heterocyclic selective serotonin reuptake inhibitors, monoamine oxidase inhibitors, and others, have been explored and found to have no effect on cocaine abstinence.[143] A pooled analysis from a multisite trial of 4 medication classes, including antidepressants, mood stabilizers, dopamine agonists, and neuroprotectives, found no significant effect on abstinence for any of the 4 classes.[144] A combined approach of newer antidepressant medication and contingency management is showing promise.[145,146]

SUMMARY

The high prevalence of stimulant abuse and its harmful consequences make the screening, diagnosis, and referral for treatment of persons with stimulant abuse a top concern for primary care providers. Having a working knowledge of use patterns, clinical symptomatology, end-organ effects, and advances in treatment of stimulant abuse is essential.

Although cocaine and amphetamine have different use patterns, duration of action, and so forth, the consequences of use are remarkably similar. Effective psychosocial treatments, for example, contingency management, are available, whereas pharmaceutical treatment remains elusive. Primary care is at the forefront of screening, brief risk reduction interventions, and diagnosis of medical sequelae, with referral to addiction specialist treatment when necessary.

ACKNOWLEDGMENTS

The author gratefully acknowledges the contributions of Nathan Sackett, RN in researching and editing sections of this article.

REFERENCES

1. Thoumi FE. Illegal drugs, economy, and society in the Andes. Washington, DC: Woodrow Wilson Center Press; 2003.
2. Spillane JF. Cocaine: from medical marvel to modern menace in the United States, 1884–1920. Baltimore (MD): Johns Hopkins University Press; 2000.
3. Musto DF. The American disease: origins of narcotic control. 3rd edition. New York: Oxford University Press; 1999.
4. Reinarman C, Levine HG, editors. Crack in America: demon drugs and social justice. Berkeley (CA): University of California Press; 1997. p. 18–51.
5. Rasmussen N. Making the first anti-depressant: amphetamine in American medicine, 1929–1950. J Hist Med Allied Sci 2006;61(3):288–323.
6. Goode E. Drugs in American society. 6th edition. New York: McGraw-Hill; 2005.
7. Hunt D, Kuck S, Truitt L. Methamphetamine use: lessons learned, final report to the National Institute of Justice 2006, February 2006 (NCJ 209730). Available at: www.ncjrs.gov/pdffiles1/nij/grants/209730.pdf. Accessed March 27, 2010.
8. Wikipedia contributors. Benzedrine. Wikipedia, The Free Encyclopedia. Available at: http://en.wikipedia.org/wiki/Benzedrine. Accessed December 20, 2010.
9. Wikipedia contributors. Amphetamine. Wikipedia, The Free Encyclopedia. Available at: http://en.wikipedia.org/wiki/Amphetamine. Accessed December 20, 2010.
10. Substance Abuse and Mental Health Services Administration. Results from the 2008 National Survey on Drug Use and Health: National findings. NSDUH Series H-36, HHS Publication No. SMA 09–4434. Rockville (MD): Office of Applied Studies; 2009.
11. Maxwell JC, Rutkowski BA. The prevalence of methamphetamine and amphetamine abuse in North America: a review of the indicators, 1992–2007. Drug Alcohol Rev 2008;27(3):229–35.
12. Substance Abuse and Mental Health Services Administration, Office of Applied Studies. Drug Abuse Warning Network, 2006: National estimates of drug-related emergency department visits. DAWN Series D-30, DHHS Publication No. (SMA) 08–4339. Rockville (MD): Department of Health and Human Services; 2008.
13. Substance Abuse and Mental Health Services Administration, Office of Applied Studies. Drug Abuse Warning Network, 2007: area profiles of drug-related mortality. HHS Publication No. SMA 09–4407, DAWN Series D-31. Rockville (MD): Department of Health and Human Services; 2009.
14. Nicosia N, Pacula RL, Kilmer B, et al. The economic cost of methamphetamine use in the United States, 2005. Santa Monica (CA): RAND Drug Policy Research Center; 2009.

15. United Nations Office on Drugs and Crime. 2009 World Drug Report. Vienna, 2009.
16. Hatsukami DK, Fischman MW. Crack cocaine and cocaine hydrochloride. Are the differences myth or reality? JAMA 1996;276(19):1580–8.
17. Urban Dictionary contributors. Cocaine. Available at: http://www. urbandictionary.com/define.php?term=cocaine. Accessed December 20, 2010.
18. Volkow ND, Wang GJ, Fischman MW, et al. Effects of route of administration on cocaine induced dopamine transporter blockade in the human brain. Life Sci 2000;67(12):1507–15.
19. US Drug Enforcement Administration. "DEA history book, 1876–1990" (drug usage & enforcement), US Department of Justice. USDoJ.gov webpage: Available at: http://www.justice.gov/dea/pubs/history/1985–1990.html. Accessed March 31, 2010.
20. US Department of Justice, National Drug Intelligence Center. National drug threat assessment 2009. Washington, DC: National Drug Intelligence Center; 2008.
21. Shesser R, Jotte R, Olshaker J. The contribution of impurities to the acute morbidity of illegal drug use. Am J Emerg Med 1991;9:336–42.
22. Kinzie E. Levamisole found in patients using cocaine. Ann Emerg Med 2009; 53(4):546–7.
23. Knowles L, Buxton JA, Skuridina N, et al. Levamisole tainted cocaine causing severe neutropenia in Alberta and British Columbia. Harm Reduct J 2009;6:30.
24. US Drug Enforcement Administration. Stats and facts. Available at: http://www. justice.gov/dea/statistics.html. Accessed April 2, 2010.
25. US Department of Justice, National Drug Intelligence Center. National methamphetamine threat assessment 2007. Washington, DC: National Drug Intelligence Center; 2006.
26. Ellenhorn MJ, Schonwald S, Ordog G, et al. Ellenhorn's medical toxicology: diagnosis and treatment of human poisoning. 2nd edition. Baltimore (MD): Williams and Wilkins; 1997.
27. Cho AK, Melega WP. Patterns of methamphetamine abuse and their consequences. J Addict Dis 2002;21(1):21–34.
28. Schifano F, Corkery JM, Cuffolo G. Smokable ("ice", "crystal meth") and non smokable amphetamine-type stimulants: clinical pharmacological and epidemiological issues, with special reference to the UK. Ann Ist Super Sanità 2007; 43(1):110–5.
29. Masand PS, Tesar GE. Use of stimulants in the medically ill. Psychiatr Clin North Am 1996;19(3):515–47.
30. Warner M. A jolt of caffeine, by the can. New York Times, November 23, 2005.
31. McCabe SE, Teter CJ, Boyd CJ. Medical use, illicit use and diversion of prescription stimulant medication. J Psychoactive Drugs 2006;38(1):43–56.
32. Volkow ND, Swanson JM. Does childhood treatment of ADHD with stimulant medication affect substance abuse in adulthood? Am J Psychiatry 2008; 165(5):553–5.
33. Sachdev M, Miller WC, Ryan T, et al. Effect of fenfluramine-derivative diet pills on cardiac valves: a meta-analysis of observational studies. Am Heart J 2002; 144(6):1065–73.
34. Kernan WN, Viscoli CM, Brass LM, et al. Phenylpropanolamine and the risk of hemorrhagic stroke. N Engl J Med 2000;343(25):1826–32.
35. Fleckenstein AE, Volz TJ, Riddle EL, et al. New insights into the mechanism of action of amphetamines. Annu Rev Pharmacol Toxicol 2007;47:681–98.

36. Howell LL, Kimmel HL. Monoamine transporters and psychostimulant addiction. Biochem Pharmacol 2008;75(1):196–217.
37. Volkow ND, Fowler JS, Wang GJ, et al. Imaging dopamine's role in drug abuse and addiction. Neuropharmacology 2009;56(Suppl 1):3–8.
38. Wee S, Carroll FI, Woolverton WL. A reduced rate of in vivo dopamine transporter binding is associated with lower relative reinforcing efficacy of stimulants. Neuropsychopharmacology 2006;31(2):351–62.
39. Chen R, Tilley MR, Wei H, et al. Abolished cocaine reward in mice with a cocaine-insensitive dopamine transporter. Proc Natl Acad Sci U S A 2006; 103(24):9333–8.
40. Caine SB, Thomsen M, Gabriel KI, et al. Lack of self-administration of cocaine in dopamine D1 receptor knock-out mice. J Neurosci 2007;27(48):13140–50.
41. Kimmel HL, O'Connor JA, Carroll FI, et al. Faster onset and dopamine transporter selectivity predict stimulant and reinforcing effects of cocaine analogs in squirrel monkeys. Pharmacol Biochem Behav 2007;86(1):45–54.
42. Kuhar MJ, Ritz MC, Boja JW. The dopamine hypothesis of the reinforcing properties of cocaine. Trends Neurosci 1991;14(7):299–302.
43. Filip M, Frankowska M, Zaniewska M, et al. The serotonergic system and its role in cocaine addiction. Pharmacol Rep 2005;57(6):685–700.
44. Rothman RB, Baumann MH, Dersch CM, et al. Amphetamine-type central nervous system stimulants release norepinephrine more potently than they release dopamine and serotonin. Synapse 2001;39(1):32–41.
45. Gass JT, Olive MF. Glutamatergic substrates of drug addiction and alcoholism. Biochem Pharmacol 2008;75(1):218–65.
46. Williams MJ, Adinoff B. The role of acetylcholine in cocaine addiction. Neuropsychopharmacology 2008;33(8):1779–97.
47. Romanelli F, Smith KM. Clinical effects and management of methamphetamine abuse. Pharmacotherapy 2006;26(8):1148–56.
48. Gorelick DA. The pharmacology of cocaine, amphetamines, and other stimulants. In: Ries RK, Fiellin DA, Miller SC, et al, editors. Principles of addiction medicine. 4th edition. Philadelphia (PA): Wolters Kluwer, Lippincott Williams and Wilkins; 2009. p. 142.
49. Hando J, Topp L, Hall W. Amphetamine-related harms and treatment preferences of regular amphetamine users in Sydney, Australia. Drug Alcohol Depend 1997;46(1–2):105–13.
50. Peck JA, Shoptaw S, Rotheram-Fuller E, et al. HIV-associated medical, behavioral, and psychiatric characteristics of treatment-seeking, methamphetamine-dependent men who have sex with men. J Addict Dis 2005;24(3):115–32.
51. O'Connor AD, Rusyniak DE, Bruno A. Cerebrovascular and cardiovascular complications of alcohol and sympathomimetic drug abuse. Med Clin North Am 2005;89(6):1343–58.
52. Gay GR. Clinical management of acute and chronic cocaine poisoning. Ann Emerg Med 1982;11(10):562–72.
53. Colfax G, Shoptaw S. The methamphetamine epidemic: implications for HIV prevention and treatment. Curr HIV/AIDS Rep 2005;2(4):194–9.
54. Myers MG, Rohsenow DJ, Monti PM, et al. Patterns of cocaine use among individuals in substance abuse treatment. Am J Drug Alcohol Abuse 1995;21(2): 223–31.
55. O'Brien CP, Gardner EL. Critical assessment of how to study addiction and its treatment: human and non-human animal models. Pharmacol Ther 2005; 108(1):18–58.

56. Kalivas PW, Pierce RC, Cornish J, et al. A role for sensitization in craving and relapse in cocaine addiction. J Psychopharmacol 1998;12(1):49–53.

57. Robinson TE, Berridge KC. The psychology and neurobiology of addiction: an incentive-sensitization view. Addiction 2000;95(Suppl 2):S91–117.

58. Bonate PL, Swann A, Silverman PB. Context-dependent cross-sensitization between cocaine and amphetamine. Life Sci 1997;60(1):PL1–7.

59. Mahoney JJ 3rd, Kalechstein AD, De La Garza R 2nd, et al. Presence and persistence of psychotic symptoms in cocaine-versus methamphetamine-dependent participants. Am J Addict 2008;17(2):83–98.

60. Fasano A, Barra A, Nicosia P, et al. Cocaine addiction: from habits to stereotypical-repetitive behaviors and punding. Drug Alcohol Depend 2008;96(1–2):178–82.

61. Hall W, Hando J, Darke S, et al. Psychological morbidity and route of administration among amphetamine users in Sydney, Australia. Addiction 1996;91(1):81–7.

62. Williamson S, Gossop M, Powis B, et al. Adverse effects of stimulant drugs in a community sample of drug users. Drug Alcohol Depend 1997;44(2–3):87–94.

63. Flaum M, Schultz SK. When does amphetamine-induced psychosis become schizophrenia? Am J Psychiatry 1996;153(6):812–5.

64. Yui K, Ishiguro T, Goto K, et al. Factors affecting the development of spontaneous recurrence of methamphetamine psychosis. Acta Psychiatr Scand 1998;97(3):220–7.

65. Mendelson JH, Sholar M, Mello NK, et al. Cocaine tolerance: behavioral, cardiovascular, and neuroendocrine function in men. Neuropsychopharmacology 1998;18(4):263–71.

66. Lim KO, Wozniak JR, Mueller BA, et al. Brain macrostructural and microstructural abnormalities in cocaine dependence. Drug Alcohol Depend 2008; 92(1–3):164–72.

67. Yucel M, Lubman DI, Solowij N, et al. Understanding drug addiction: a neuropsychological perspective. Aust N Z J Psychiatry 2007;41(12):957–68.

68. Coffey SF, Dansky BS, Carrigan MH, et al. Acute and protracted cocaine abstinence in an outpatient population: a prospective study of mood, sleep and withdrawal symptoms. Drug Alcohol Depend 2000;59(3):277–86.

69. Lago JA, Kosten TR. Stimulant withdrawal. Addiction 1994;89(11):1477–81.

70. Anthony JC, Warner LA, Kessler RC. Comparitive epidemiology of dependence on tobacco, alcohol, controlled substances, and inhalants: basic findings from the National Comorbidity Survey. Exp Clin Psychopharmacol 1994;2:244–68.

71. Woody GE, Cottler LB, Cacciola J. Severity of dependence: data from the DSM-IV field trials. Addiction 1993;88(11):1573–9.

72. Gossop M, Griffiths P, Powis B, et al. Cocaine: patterns of use, route of administration, and severity of dependence. Br J Psychiatry 1994;164(5):660–4.

73. Gorelick DA. The rate hypothesis and agonist substitution approaches to cocaine abuse treatment. Adv Pharmacol 1998;42:995–7.

74. Association AP. Diagnostic and statistical manual of mental disorders. Text Revision. 4th edition. Washington, DC: American Psychiatric Association; 2000.

75. Agrawal A, Lynskey MT. Are there genetic influences on addiction: evidence from family, adoption and twin studies. Addiction 2008;103(7):1069–81.

76. Boghdadi MS, Henning RJ. Cocaine: pathophysiology and clinical toxicology. Heart Lung 1997;26(6):466–83 [quiz: 484–5].

77. Qureshi AI, Suri MF, Guterman LR, et al. Cocaine use and the likelihood of nonfatal myocardial infarction and stroke: data from the Third National Health and Nutrition Examination Survey. Circulation 2001;103(4):502–6.

78. Gitman MD, Singhal PC. Cocaine-induced renal disease. Expert Opin Drug Saf 2004;3(5):441–8.
79. Glauser J, Queen JR. An overview of non-cardiac cocaine toxicity. J Emerg Med 2007;32(2):181–6.
80. Doctora JS, Williams CW, Bennett CR, et al. Rhabdomyolysis in the acutely cocaine-intoxicated patient sustaining maxillofacial trauma: report of a case and review of the literature. J Oral Maxillofac Surg 2003; 61(8):964–7.
81. Goodger NM, Wang J, Pogrel MA. Palatal and nasal necrosis resulting from cocaine misuse. Br Dent J 2005;198(6):333–4.
82. Kuczkowski KM. The effects of drug abuse on pregnancy. Curr Opin Obstet Gynecol 2007;19(6):578–85.
83. Phupong V, Darojn D. Amphetamine abuse in pregnancy: the impact on obstetric outcome. Arch Gynecol Obstet 2007;276(2):167–70.
84. Williams JH, Ross L. Consequences of prenatal toxin exposure for mental health in children and adolescents: a systematic review. Eur Child Adolesc Psychiatry 2007;16(4):243–53.
85. Neiman J, Haapaniemi HM, Hillbom M. Neurological complications of drug abuse: pathophysiological mechanisms. Eur J Neurol 2000;7(6):595–606.
86. Warner EA. Cocaine abuse. Ann Intern Med 1993;119(3):226–35.
87. Harris D, Batki SL. Stimulant psychosis: symptom profile and acute clinical course. Am J Addict 2000;9(1):28–37.
88. Featherstone RE, Kapur S, Fletcher PJ. The amphetamine-induced sensitized state as a model of schizophrenia. Prog Neuropsychopharmacol Biol Psychiatry 2007;31(8):1556–71.
89. Buffenstein A, Heaster J, Ko P. Chronic psychotic illness from methamphetamine. Am J Psychiatry 1999;156(4):662.
90. Mello NK, Mendelson JH. Cocaine's effects on neuroendocrine systems: clinical and preclinical studies. Pharmacol Biochem Behav 1997;57(3):571–99.
91. Carey JC. Pharmacological effects on sexual function. Obstet Gynecol Clin North Am 2006;33(4):599–620.
92. Afonso L, Mohammad T, Thatai D. Crack whips the heart: a review of the cardiovascular toxicity of cocaine. Am J Cardiol 2007;100(6):1040–3.
93. Lange RA, Hillis LD. Cardiovascular complications of cocaine use. N Engl J Med 2001;345(5):351–8.
94. Yeo KK, Wijetunga M, Ito H, et al. The association of methamphetamine use and cardiomyopathy in young patients. Am J Med 2007;120(2):165–71.
95. Tashkin DP. Airway effects of marijuana, cocaine, and other inhaled illicit agents. Curr Opin Pulm Med 2001;7(2):43–61.
96. Wolff AJ, O'Donnell AE. Pulmonary effects of illicit drug use. Clin Chest Med 2004;25(1):203–16.
97. Shoptaw S. Methamphetamine use in urban gay and bisexual populations. Top HIV Med 2006;14(2):84–7.
98. Des Jarlais DC, Friedman SR. HIV infection among intravenous drug users: epidemiology and risk reduction. AIDS 1987;1(2):67–76.
99. Chaisson RE, Bacchetti P, Osmond D, et al. Cocaine use and HIV infection in intravenous drug users in San Francisco. JAMA 1989;261(4):561–5.
100. Hahn JA, Page-Shafer K, Lum PJ, et al. Hepatitis C virus seroconversion among young injection drug users: relationships and risks. J Infect Dis 2002;186(11): 1558–64.

101. Booth RE, Watters JK, Chitwood DD. HIV risk-related sex behaviors among injection drug users, crack smokers, and injection drug users who smoke crack. Am J Public Health 1993;83(8):1144–8.
102. Edlin BR, Irwin KL, Faruque S, et al. Intersecting epidemics—crack cocaine use and HIV infection among inner-city young adults. Multicenter Crack Cocaine and HIV Infection Study Team. N Engl J Med 1994;331(21): 1422–7.
103. Fisher DG, Reynolds GL, Napper LE. Use of crystal methamphetamine, Viagra, and sexual behavior. Curr Opin Infect Dis 2010;23(1):53–6.
104. Stall R, Paul JP, Greenwood G, et al. Alcohol use, drug use and alcohol-related problems among men who have sex with men: the Urban Men's Health Study. Addiction 2001;96(11):1589–601.
105. Colfax G, Coates TJ, Husnik MJ, et al. Longitudinal patterns of methamphetamine, popper (amyl nitrite), and cocaine use and high-risk sexual behavior among a cohort of San Francisco men who have sex with men. J Urban Health 2005;82(1 Suppl 1):i62–70.
106. Halkitis PN, Mukherjee PP, Palamar JJ. Longitudinal modeling of methamphetamine use and sexual risk behaviors in gay and bisexual men. AIDS Behav 2009;13(4):783–91.
107. Thiede H, Jenkins RA, Carey JW, et al. Determinants of recent HIV infection among Seattle-area men who have sex with men. Am J Public Health 2009; 99(Suppl 1):S157–64.
108. Semple SJ, Strathdee SA, Zians J, et al. Sexual risk behavior associated with co-administration of methamphetamine and other drugs in a sample of HIV-positive men who have sex with men. Am J Addict 2009;18(1):65–72.
109. Prestage G, Jin F, Kippax S, et al. Use of illicit drugs and erectile dysfunction medications and subsequent HIV infection among gay men in Sydney, Australia. J Sex Med 2009;6(8):2311–20.
110. Sanchez TH, Gallagher KM. Factors associated with recent sildenafil (Viagra) use among men who have sex with men in the United States. J Acquir Immune Defic Syndr 2006;42(1):95–100.
111. Ostrow DG, Plankey MW, Cox C, et al. Specific sex drug combinations contribute to the majority of recent HIV seroconversions among MSM in the MACS. J Acquir Immune Defic Syndr 2009;51(3):349–55.
112. Screening and Behavioral Counseling Interventions in Primary Care to Reduce Alcohol Misuse, Topic Page. April 2004. U.S. Preventive Services Task Force. http://www.uspreventiveservicestaskforce.org/uspstf/uspsdrin.htm. Accessed November 23, 2010.
113. Screening for Illicit Drug Use, Topic Page. January 2008. U.S. Preventive Services Task Force. Available at: http://www.uspreventiveservicestaskforce.org/uspstf/uspsdrug.htm. Accessed December 17, 2010.
114. Kulig JW. Tobacco, alcohol, and other drugs: the role of the pediatrician in prevention, identification, and management of substance abuse. Pediatrics 2005;115(3):816–21.
115. Guidelines for women's health care. 2nd edition. Washington, DC: American College of Obstetricians and Gynecologists; 2002.
116. Center for Substance Abuse Treatment. A guide to substance abuse services for primary care clinicians. Treatment Improvement Protocol (TIP) Series, Number 24. DHHS Pub. No. (SMA) 97-3139. Washington, DC: US Government Printing Office; 1997.

117. Smith PC, Schmidt SM, Allensworth-Davies D, et al. A single-question screening test for drug use in primary care. Arch Intern Med 2010;170(13):1155–60.

118. Center for Substance Abuse Treatment. Brief interventions and brief therapies for substance abuse. Treatment Improvement Protocol (TIP) Series, Number 34. DHHS Pub. No. (SMA) 99-3353. Washington, DC: US Government Printing Office; 1999.

119. Bertholet N, Daeppen JB, Wietlisbach V, et al. Reduction of alcohol consumption by brief alcohol intervention in primary care: systematic review and meta-analysis. Arch Intern Med 2005;165(9):986–95.

120. Kaner EF, Beyer F, Dickinson HO, et al. Effectiveness of brief alcohol interventions in primary care populations. Cochrane Database Syst Rev 2007;2: CD004148.

121. Whitlock EP, Polen MR, Green CA, et al. Behavioral counseling interventions in primary care to reduce risky/harmful alcohol use by adults: a summary of the evidence for the U.S. Preventive Services Task Force. Ann Intern Med 2004; 140(7):557–68.

122. Madras BK, Compton WM, Avula D, et al. Screening, brief interventions, referral to treatment (SBIRT) for illicit drug and alcohol use at multiple healthcare sites: comparison at intake and 6 months later. Drug Alcohol Depend 2009;99(1–3): 280–95.

123. Bernstein J, Bernstein E, Tassiopoulos K, et al. Brief motivational intervention at a clinic visit reduces cocaine and heroin use. Drug Alcohol Depend 2005;77(1): 49–59.

124. Baker A, Lee NK, Claire M, et al. Brief cognitive behavioural interventions for regular amphetamine users: a step in the right direction. Addiction 2005; 100(3):367–78.

125. Vocci FJ, Montoya ID. Psychological treatments for stimulant misuse, comparing and contrasting those for amphetamine dependence and those for cocaine dependence. Curr Opin Psychiatry 2009;22(3):263–8.

126. Dutra L, Stathopoulou G, Basden SL, et al. A meta-analytic review of psychosocial interventions for substance use disorders. Am J Psychiatry 2008;165(2): 179–87.

127. Carroll KM, Nich C, Ball SA, et al. Treatment of cocaine and alcohol dependence with psychotherapy and disulfiram. Addiction 1998;93(5):713–27.

128. Maude-Griffin PM, Hohenstein JM, Humfleet GL, et al. Superior efficacy of cognitive-behavioral therapy for urban crack cocaine abusers: main and matching effects. J Consult Clin Psychol 1998;66(5):832–7.

129. Monti PM, Rohsenow DJ, Michalec E, et al. Brief coping skills treatment for cocaine abuse: substance use outcomes at three months. Addiction 1997; 92(12):1717–28.

130. Carroll KM, Rounsaville BJ, Gawin FH. A comparative trial of psychotherapies for ambulatory cocaine abusers: relapse prevention and interpersonal psychotherapy. Am J Drug Alcohol Abuse 1991;17(3):229–47.

131. Lee NK, Rawson RA. A systematic review of cognitive and behavioural therapies for methamphetamine dependence. Drug Alcohol Rev 2008;27(3): 309–17.

132. Higgins ST, Tidey JW, Rogers RE. Contingency management and the community reinforcement approach. In: Ries RK, Fiellin DA, Miller SC, et al, editors. Principles of addiction medicine. 4th edition. Philadelphia (PA): Wolters Kluwer, Lippincott Williams and Wilkins; 2009. p. 787, 788.

133. Griffith JD, Rowan-Szal GA, Roark RR, et al. Contingency management in outpatient methadone treatment: a meta-analysis. Drug Alcohol Depend 2000; 58(1–2):55–66.

134. Lussier JP, Heil SH, Mongeon JA, et al. A meta-analysis of voucher-based reinforcement therapy for substance use disorders. Addiction 2006;101(2): 192–203.

135. Prendergast ML, Podus D, Chang E, et al. The effectiveness of drug abuse treatment: a meta-analysis of comparison group studies. Drug Alcohol Depend 2002;67(1):53–72.

136. Epstein DH, Hawkins WE, Covi L, et al. Cognitive-behavioral therapy plus contingency management for cocaine use: findings during treatment and across 12-month follow-up. Psychol Addict Behav 2003;17(1):73–82.

137. Higgins ST, Wong CJ, Badger GJ, et al. Contingent reinforcement increases cocaine abstinence during outpatient treatment and 1 year of follow-up. J Consult Clin Psychol 2000;68(1):64–72.

138. Petry NM, Alessi SM, Hanson T. Contingency management improves abstinence and quality of life in cocaine abusers. J Consult Clin Psychol 2007;75(2):307–15.

139. Secades-Villa R, Garcia-Rodriguez O, Higgins ST, et al. Community reinforcement approach plus vouchers for cocaine dependence in a community setting in Spain: six-month outcomes. J Subst Abuse Treat 2008;34(2):202–7.

140. Rawson RA, McCann MJ, Flammino F, et al. A comparison of contingency management and cognitive-behavioral approaches for stimulant-dependent individuals. Addiction 2006;101(2):267–74.

141. Roll JM, Petry NM, Stitzer ML, et al. Contingency management for the treatment of methamphetamine use disorders. Am J Psychiatry 2006;163(11):1993–9.

142. Shoptaw S, Reback CJ, Peck JA, et al. Behavioral treatment approaches for methamphetamine dependence and HIV-related sexual risk behaviors among urban gay and bisexual men. Drug Alcohol Depend 2005;78(2):125–34.

143. Lima MS, Reisser AA, Soares BG, et al. Antidepressants for cocaine dependence. Cochrane Database Syst Rev 2003;2:CD002950.

144. Elkashef A, Holmes TH, Bloch DA, et al. Retrospective analyses of pooled data from CREST I and CREST II trials for treatment of cocaine dependence. Addiction 2005;100(Suppl 1):91–101.

145. Moeller FG, Schmitz JM, Steinberg JL, et al. Citalopram combined with behavioral therapy reduces cocaine use: a double-blind, placebo-controlled trial. Am J Drug Alcohol Abuse 2007;33(3):367–78.

146. Poling J, Oliveto A, Petry N, et al. Six-month trial of bupropion with contingency management for cocaine dependence in a methadone-maintained population. Arch Gen Psychiatry 2006;63(2):219–28.

Opioid Dependence

Joseph J. Benich III, MD

KEYWORDS

- Opioid • Dependence • Withdrawal • Detoxification
- Methadone • Buprenorphine

Key Points	
Clinical Recommendations	**Level of Evidence**
Opioid dependence can be effectively managed using methadone or buprenorphine in maintenance therapy treatment	A
If other factors such as treatment availability are equivalent, methadone should be used preferentially over buprenorphine to manage opioid dependence	A
Detoxification treatment alone is inferior to maintenance treatment using methadone or buprenorphine	B
Treatment programs using psychosocial interventions in conjunction with pharmacologic therapy have resulted in higher rates of treatment adherence and abstinence from opioid use	B

EPIDEMIOLOGY

The estimated prevalence of opioid dependence in adults in the United States was 898,000 in 2005.[1] Men are more likely than women to have opioid-related disorders, and people who are opioid dependent have a higher frequency of antisocial personality disorders than individuals in the general population.[2] It has been shown that more than half of the patients seeking treatment of opioid dependency have coexisting psychiatric conditions.[3] Depression and posttraumatic stress disorder have especially high concordance rates with this condition out of the axis I disorders.[4]

Opioid-dependent individuals have an increased likelihood of using multiple drugs at the same time.[5] In particular, nicotine and opioid dependence go hand in hand, with about 9 out of every 10 opioid-dependent persons also meeting criteria for nicotine dependence.[4] Dependence on opioids leads to many health and social problems

Department of Family Medicine, Medical University of South Carolina, 295 Calhoun Street, Charleston, SC 29425, USA
E-mail address: benichjj@musc.edu

Prim Care Clin Office Pract 38 (2011) 59–70
doi:10.1016/j.pop.2010.11.005   **primarycare.theclinics.com**
0095-4543/11/$ – see front matter © 2011 Elsevier Inc. All rights reserved.

for individuals. Regular opioid use has been linked to increased rates of human immunodeficiency virus (HIV) infection, crime, mortality, and unemployment.[6] These individual issues in turn lead to societal health concerns and increased costs. Opioid dependence results in lost productivity for affected individuals in addition to being associated with higher law enforcement and health care costs for the community at large.[7]

Most people who are opioid dependent do not receive a structured treatment of their disorder. About 337,000 people entered treatment programs for opioid dependence in 2007.[8] Treatment is now provided in both methadone clinics and office-based programs coordinated and run by outpatient physicians.

PHARMACOLOGY

The alkaloid morphine is the principal active ingredient in opioids. These drugs act by binding to receptors on the cell membranes, especially in the central nervous system. There are multiple opioid receptor subtypes, including μ, δ, κ, and λ. Endorphins, endogenous opioids, take part in the regulation of inherent behaviors, such as survival instincts, through stimulation of these receptors.[9] Triggering opioid receptors can affect multiple systems influencing pain, mood, respiration, blood pressure, and gastrointestinal function. Exogenous drugs that act through the same receptors as those which are stimulated by endorphins are defined as opioids. Regardless of whether the activating chemical is synthetic or natural, receptor activation has been connected to the conditioning of rewarding stimuli.[10]

Opioid drugs are primarily categorized and defined according to their capacity to bind to and activate the different opioid receptor types. Agonists bind and activate receptors, whereas antagonists bind but do not activate receptors.[11] There are also partial agonists and antagonists. Opioids can have profound effects on pain and the anticipation of pain.[12] They can also affect mood and feeling, thereby causing a sense of tranquility, decreased anxiety, and sleepiness. Individuals can have very different responses to these medications. Everything from a sense of euphoria or rush to nausea, vomiting, and depression of respiration can be seen with the use of this class of drugs.[13]

Neurobiological changes play a role in the progression of opioid dependence. The locus coeruleus is the region of the brain that contains the main grouping of norepinephrine-containing neurons. It has been shown that norepinephrine may play a role in encouraging drug-seeking behaviors and eventual dependence.[14] The locus coeruleus is the primary source of almost all noradrenergic afferents in the brain. Different opioids can invoke separate responses in reward centers in this and other regions of the medial forebrain. Opioid stimulation can proportionately affect the magnitude of a reward by potentiating the release of neurotransmitters.[15] For example, dopamine is a neurotransmitter that seems to strengthen the inherent rewarding characteristics of drugs of abuse.[16] Some receptor activation can produce effects through negative feedback too. Opioid μ agonists inhibit the activity of the locus coeruleus. The opioid withdrawal syndrome is believed to be largely because of hyperactivity in the locus coeruleus once this inhibition is discontinued.[17] Changes in G protein–coupled receptors, variations in transcription and translation, and increased activity of cyclic adenosine monophosphate second messenger channels also contribute to withdrawal and tolerance.[18]

Treatment options for opioid dependence include opioid replacement programs. Methadone and buprenorphine are 2 of the drugs used for treatment. Nonopioid medications, such as clonidine and lofexidine, are also used with these drugs to help control symptoms of withdrawal.[19] These α_2-adrenergic medications are typically used for the treatment of hypertension, but they are also effectively used for controlling opioid withdrawal symptoms. These medications decrease some of the aforementioned noradrenergic hyperactivity in the central nervous system to achieve the symptom reduction.[19] Although methadone and buprenorphine are both used for treatment, they have different mechanisms of action at the opioid receptors. Buprenorphine is a partial μ receptor agonist that also possesses some antagonist properties at the κ receptor.[20] Buprenorphine is often combined with naloxone, an opioid receptor antagonist, to prevent abuse through injection of the medication that is intended to be used sublingually. This combination is effective because naloxone has minimal efficacy when taken sublingually, but it exerts full antagonist properties if injected.[21] Because it is only a partial agonist, buprenorphine has a lower threshold for the euphoric effects it can induce when compared with full agonists.[22] On the other hand, methadone is a full agonist that primarily activates the same opioid μ receptors, but it does not reach a similar threshold. Full agonists are controlled substances because they can produce effects similar to the drugs of abuse they are used to replace. The half-lives of both methadone and buprenorphine allow them to be used in a daily dosing regimen.

DEPENDENCE

Substance dependence is present when an individual continues to use a substance despite experiencing several problems directly stemming from its use. Dependence is manifested by a combination of behavioral, cognitive, and physiologic symptoms and typically leads to compulsive drug-taking behavior, tolerance, and withdrawal. It should be pointed out that although tolerance and withdrawal are part of the diagnostic criteria, they are not necessary components of a diagnosis of substance dependence. Of the 7 major criteria, 3 or more need to be present in the same 12-month period to make the diagnosis of substance dependence. The 7 criteria are as follows: (1) tolerance; (2) withdrawal; (3) unintentional overuse with regard to duration or amount; (4) inability to reduce use despite wanting to do so; (5) inordinate amounts of time dedicated to use, acquisition, or recuperation of the substance; (6) other important life activities sacrificed in lieu of use; and (7) continued use of a substance despite the knowledge that its use is likely causing or exacerbating health or mental issues.[23]

Opioid dependence can be a challenging issue to identify and manage. Individuals are not always candid about their substance use. Anyone can develop an opioid-use disorder. However, there are at least 3 major populations of individuals who seem to be at an increased risk of becoming dependent or who are at a minimum at increased risk for misuse that can lead to dependence. The groups are those who purchase street drugs to achieve the euphoric high from abusing them, people who work in health care professions, and people who are on chronic pain medications because of their chronic pain syndromes.[24] Patients undergoing chronic pain therapy should be closely monitored. The use of opioids needs to be only one component of a complete management plan that includes other modalities such as physical therapy, behavior-modification techniques, and counseling about realistic expectations. Individuals in the medical field, such as doctors, nurses, and pharmacists, are at increased risk because of easier access to opioid medications. The third group typically uses opioids frequently enough to put themselves in the high-risk category for becoming dependent.[24] Physicians should be on the lookout for drug-seeking behaviors or signs of relapse in patients who were known to be former opioid addicts.

Concerning signals in such patients include looking for early narcotic prescription refills, going to multiple physicians to obtain restricted medications, having urine drug screens inconsistent with medications currently prescribed to them, and demanding replacement medications or higher doses.[2]

It deserves mentioning that the American Psychiatric Association is presently planning to release the Diagnostic and Statistical Manual of Mental Disorders V in 2013. Changes relevant to this topic include a proposed reorganization of current categories of substance use. A new category termed opioid-use disorder would encompass the current categories of opioid abuse and opioid dependence. The term dependence would only be used in reference to physiologic dependence. Other proposed specifiers would further delineate the severity of opioid-use disorder into categories, such as moderate or severe, based on the number of positive criteria satisfied by an individual. Further classification would also provide terminology for stages of remission.

WITHDRAWAL

Many individuals with opioid dependence develop withdrawal if they discontinue use. This withdrawal seems to clearly stem from most abusers developing high levels of tolerance.[23] Withdrawal symptoms typically start somewhere around 8 to 16 hours after discontinuation of the opioid in dependent individuals. This timeframe seems to best apply to discontinuation of drugs with shorter half-lives, such as morphine or heroin. The worst symptoms usually reach maximal intensity around 36 to 72 hours after cessation of use. Although the primary withdrawal syndrome typically lasts 5 to 8 days, a protracted period may follow with milder symptoms.[24] During the prolonged phase after drug cessation, an individual may experience multiple general unpleasant symptoms for months, such as trouble in sleeping, unprovoked irritability, and variations in pain tolerance.[24] Acute opioid withdrawal symptoms involve multiple systems in the body. Symptoms vary in individuals but can include the following: yawning, nausea, vomiting, diarrhea, rhinorrhea, tachycardia, piloerection, pupillary dilatation, hypertension, lacrimation, fever, insomnia, irritability, craving, and restlessness.[25] Acute- or prolonged-phase cravings may be responsible for frequent relapses.

When withdrawal is identified in the clinical setting, management should be initiated promptly. General supportive measures include good nutrition and a safe environment for the patient. An individual should also be allowed adequate time to rest during this period. Complete discontinuation is not recommended because of the severity of symptoms experienced by these patients, including high levels of anxiety. The best approach is typically to replace the chronically used opioid with long-acting opioid agonists to reduce the severity of withdrawal symptoms.[26] Patients do not need to be hospitalized for this process when they are otherwise medically stable. Other medications that can be used to control symptoms include antiemetics for nausea, muscle relaxants to reduce spasms, nonsteroidal antiinflammatory drugs to reduce pain, antidiarrheal drugs, and sleeping aides such as trazodone with lower abuse potential.

DETOXIFICATION

Detoxification involves the pharmacologic management of opioid withdrawal. The objective of detoxification is to facilitate the discontinuation of opioid use in a controlled manner that minimizes unpleasant symptoms and achieves long-term success rates with regard to program retention and continued drug abstinence.[26] Detoxification alone is not typically considered a successful treatment option for opioid dependence, but it is usually a necessary step to allow for long-term abstinence-based treatment programs.[27] Short-term detoxification takes place in a period of fewer than 30 days, and long-term detoxification lasts somewhere between 31 and 180 days. Detoxification performed gradually is generally more effective than a sudden discontinuation of opioids.[28]

Detoxification is typically achieved through 1 of the 2 basic regimens, tapering using a long-acting agonist such as methadone or abrupt cessation of opioid use while managing symptoms with medications such as clonidine. The latter method can be induced through the use of an antagonist, such as naloxone, which can limit the length of the withdrawal period but can increase the severity of withdrawal symptoms. This technique of using both opioid antagonists and symptom-controlling medications is referred to as rapid opioid detoxification.[29] Another version called ultrarapid or ultra-short detoxification was developed, whereby patients are anesthetized, intubated, and mechanically ventilated. A large dose of an antagonist is then administered while the patient is unconscious to hasten the withdrawal phase. The ultrarapid detoxification method has been shown to reduce the duration of withdrawal symptoms compared with methadone taper techniques.[30] However, severe complications have been experienced by patients undergoing ultrarapid detoxification.[31] Also, a randomized trial did not show any advantage of anesthesia-assisted detoxification over detoxification using clonidine or buprenorphine. Results from this trial showed no statistically significant difference in completion of inpatient and 12-week treatment programs among the 3 treatment groups.[32] A systematic review also supported the conclusion that the high economic cost and risks of serious complications associated with anesthesia-mediated detoxification outweigh potential benefits. More specifically, increased rates of respiratory and cardiac arrests were observed in detoxification methods using anesthesia or heavy sedation.[33] Therefore, pharmacologic detoxification not using anesthesia or heavy sedation is supported by the literature as being beneficial for patients. Patients who have low levels of dependence on opioids or who have been addicted for a short period of time typically warrant an attempt at detoxification.[34]

PHYSICIAN REQUIREMENTS TO PRESCRIBE MAINTENANCE MEDICATIONS

Physicians were given the option of conducting office-based treatment of opioid addiction by the Drug and Addiction Treatment Act of 2000.[35] This act allows qualifying physicians to receive a waiver to practice medication-assisted opioid addiction therapy with Schedule III, IV, or V narcotic medications specifically approved by the Food and Drug Administration for this purpose. Buprenorphine tablets as well as buprenorphine/naloxone combination tablets received such approval in 2002. As part of the qualification process, physicians must notify the Center for Substance Abuse Treatment of their intent to practice using these medications to treat opioid-dependent patients before actually prescribing them. Stipulations include a physician not treating more than 30 patients at a time in the first year and an ability to refer these patients for appropriate counseling and nonpharmacologic therapies. The limit can be raised to 100 patients after the initial year through another notification and approval process. The Drug Enforcement Administration (DEA) assigns each doctor a special identification number that needs to be included on all buprenorphine prescriptions. A licensed physician must meet any one or more of the following criteria to qualify for a waiver: (1) board certified in addiction psychiatry from the American Board of Medical Specialties; (2) certified in addiction medicine from the American Society of Addiction Medicine; (3) board certified in addiction medicine from the American Osteopathic Association; (4) completed at least 8 hours of training dealing with the treatment and management of opioid-addicted patients, which is provided by a permitted organization; (5) participated as an investigator in clinical trials resulting in approval of a narcotic drug used for maintenance or detoxification treatment; or (6) completed training or exhibited experience demonstrating an ability to treat and manage opioid-dependent patients as deemed satisfactory by the physician's state medical licensing board.[36] Registration and training information is available online at buprenorphine.samhsa.gov.

MAINTENANCE THERAPY

Although detoxification has been successful in select patient populations trying to eliminate the use of all opioids, good quality evidence supports that detoxification is inferior compared with ongoing, aka maintenance, medication treatment with either buprenorphine or methadone. Study results have demonstrated that patients who stay in maintenance treatment programs longer have been able to achieve lengthier periods of abstinence from illicit drug use.[37] Maintenance therapy has also been shown to be superior to abstinence therapy with regard to achieving longer retention rates in treatment programs and reducing illegal drug use.[38] Similar results were demonstrated when buprenorphine was used as the maintenance medication. A trial comparing buprenorphine maintenance therapy to detoxification showed superior retention rates in the maintenance group at 1 year.[39]

Methadone

Traditionally, methadone is dispensed and managed in dedicated clinics that focus on opioid dependence therapy and incorporate a wide array of ancillary services. Patient criteria for methadone therapy include being 18 years or older and demonstrating physiologic opioid dependence for at least 1 year. Full office-based treatment with methadone is an option, but the rigorous federal and state requirements that must be met by physicians and patients make this a less-popular option.[2] A modified version of this treatment regimen has been available since 2000, whereby physicians may provide methadone to patients as part of an overall maintenance treatment plan. These patients are typically referred from standard methadone clinics after demonstrating 3 years of stable compliance with methadone maintenance therapy.[2] Criteria that seem to suggest potential success of an individual receiving office-based opioid-agonist maintenance therapy include first receiving 1 to 5 years of methadone from a dedicated clinic, a recent track record of negative urine drug screen results, no untreated psychiatric conditions, no illegal activity, and an ability to sustain financial support.[40]

Methadone dosing usually starts around 20 to 30 mg/d, and the dose is titrated up based on the severity of a patient's withdrawal symptoms. A maintenance dose is considered satisfactory once symptoms are controlled for at least 24 hours. Methadone has a long half-life, so it may take up to 10 days to find a steady-state maintenance dose.[2] Methadone pharmacotherapy continued for more than 180 days in duration meets the criteria for maintenance therapy. If methadone is used for lesser than 180 days, then detoxification is considered to occur. Maintenance therapy may be slowly tapered off over months to years, or patients may choose to stay on a stable dose indefinitely. Studies suggest that patients have better outcomes when maintained on higher methadone doses, for example, 80 to 100 mg/d, rather than lower doses.[41] Other benefits exist from controlling opioid dependence with methadone. Maintenance therapy has been shown to effectively reduce the spread of HIV among opioid-dependent individuals.[42]

Side effects of chronic methadone therapy include constipation, sexual side effects such as erectile dysfunction or decreased libido, excessive diaphoresis, fatigue, respiratory depression, and peripheral edema. Methadone use has also been linked with concerning cardiac outcomes. Regular use can be associated with QTc interval prolongation and torsades de pointes.[43] It has also been shown that methadone use may increase the risk for sudden cardiac death.[44] Methadone now carries a black-box warning regarding its proarrhythmic potential. An independent panel of experts met in 2008 and made the following recommendations regarding regular methadone use: (1) patients should be informed of the risk of arrhythmia, (2) patients should be screened for pertinent cardiac history, (3) ECG monitoring should be performed, and (4) reductions in dose or even discontinuation of use should be considered if QTc interval prolongation is observed.[45]

Buprenorphine

Treatment with buprenorphine/naloxone has 3 phases termed induction, stabilization, and maintenance. Therapy should generally start 12 to 24 hours after cessation of short-acting opioid use or 24 to 48 hours after discontinuing use of long-acting opioids. The induction phase typically lasts 3 to 7 days. Day 1 consists of starting with a 4/1 mg dose of the medication followed by a second dose 2 hours later if withdrawal symptoms persist. Over the next 6 days, this dose is titrated up to a maximum of 32/8 mg/d. The stabilization phase then begins and usually lasts 1 to 2 months. The goal of this stage of therapy is to find the minimal effective dose to decrease cravings, eliminate withdrawal, and minimize side effects of buprenorphine/naloxone. Most patients require a daily dose of at least 12/3 mg of buprenorphine/naloxone to achieve these goals. Maintenance therapy is indefinite and focuses on monitoring for illicit drug use, minimizing cravings, and avoiding triggers to use.[1]

Individual studies have shown that buprenorphine can reduce illicit opioid use with long-term therapy.[39] Literature reviews have confirmed the efficacy of buprenorphine compared with placebo with regard to treatment retention and reduced use of illicit drugs.[46] Side effects of buprenorphine include respiratory depression, headache, sleepiness, constipation, and urinary retention. However, studies have reflected high patient satisfaction with buprenorphine/naloxone therapy in a primary care setting.[47]

Methadone versus Buprenorphine

The National Guideline Clearinghouse recommendations state that both methadone and buprenorphine are recommended options for the management of opioid dependence when using flexible dosing regimens of oral formulations. Whether methadone or buprenorphine is a better treatment option needs to be determined on a case-by-case basis. Factors to consider when choosing a maintenance medication include a physician's individualized estimations of risks and benefits for treatment with each medication, the person's history of opioid dependence, and the patient's commitment to a long-term management strategy. If the evaluation process finds both pharmacotherapy options to be equally suitable for an individual, then the clearinghouse recommends methadone as the first choice. Regardless of which medication is chosen, daily dose administration is recommended for at least the first 3 months of treatment and until a patient's compliance can be reasonably assured. The last portion of the recommendations emphasize that agonist maintenance therapy should only be used as one component of an entire supportive care program.[48]

Head-to-head comparison studies have shown that methadone maintenance results in longer treatment retention than buprenorphine.[49] However, results vary with dose dependence of the patients receiving therapy. Treatment with buprenorphine has been shown to be equivocal to methadone therapy when doses of less than 40 mg are required.[50] Methadone maintenance may not be as safe as buprenorphine when taking into consideration the possibility of medication diversion because treatment doses of methadone are likely lethal for opioid-naive individuals, whereas those of buprenorphine are not.[51] Also, buprenorphine seems to have a ceiling effect for respiratory depression, whereas methadone's full-opioid agonist properties lead to more respiratory depression with increasing doses of methadone.[52] Cost can play a factor in treatment feasibility. A study that compared the cost of different maintenance treatment options found that clinic-based methadone therapy was less expensive than office-based treatment with either methadone or buprenorphine.[53] In general, methadone treatment is less expensive than programs using buprenorphine. The bottom line is that pharmacologic maintenance treatments are preferable to no treatment, and patients have fewer negative outcomes when they remain in treatment longer.

NONPHARMACOLOGIC THERAPY

Nonpharmacologic therapy for opioid dependence can be an important adjunct to medication-based treatment plans and can also be an effective standalone treatment option. When compared with pharmacologic treatment alone, treatment programs using psychosocial interventions in conjunction with pharmacologic therapy have resulted in higher rates of treatment adherence and abstinence from opioid use at follow-up evaluations.[34] Some examples of psychosocial interventions are contingency management, biofeedback, family therapy, community reinforcement, 12-step groups, and cognitive-behavioral therapy. Individual studies have shown benefit from inclusion of such interventions. A study conducted in the primary care setting demonstrated a positive association between treatment retention and counseling attendance.[54] However, systematic reviews have found drawing conclusions about psychosocial interventions compared with pharmacologic therapy difficult because of the multitude of interventions used in various individual studies.[55]

The Narcotics Anonymous is an example of a 12-step self-help group that has been shown to improve rehabilitation outcomes. Studies investigating the effects of participation in the Narcotics Anonymous have found improved drug-using outcomes for opioid-dependent individuals who attend group meetings.[56] It has also been shown that a positive correlation exists between the duration of time attending the Narcotics Anonymous meetings and the duration of abstinence from illicit drug use.[57] A 5-year follow-up study found that abstinence from opiates increased throughout the duration of the study and that individuals who had attended the Narcotics Anonymous meetings were more likely to be abstinent when compared with those who did not have abstinence-based therapy.[58]

SUMMARY

Opioid dependence is becoming more prevalent in the United States, especially through increased use of prescription opioids. This condition results in high costs and health concerns for individual users and the society at large. Opioid dependence presents a challenging issue for physicians to identify and treat. Managing withdrawal symptoms is an important component of treatment, which can be accomplished with a wide array of medications. Therapy options to treat dependence include detoxification, nonpharmacologic treatment plans, and maintenance replacement treatment with either methadone or buprenorphine. Methadone has been shown to be more effective than buprenorphine, especially in patients requiring higher doses of replacement medications. However, buprenorphine therapy is also affective and can be conducted in the outpatient setting with less-stringent restrictions by physicians meeting necessary requirements. A combination of maintenance replacement therapy and nonpharmacologic interventions seems to maximize therapeutic efficacy in achieving abstinence from opioids.

REFERENCES

1. Donaher PA, Welsh C. Managing opioid addiction with buprenorphine. Am Fam Physician 2006;73(9):1573–8.
2. Krambeer LL, Von McKnelly W, Gabrielli, et al. Methadone therapy for opioid dependence. Am Fam Physician 2001;63:2404–10.
3. Brooner RK, King VL, Kidorf M, et al. Psychiatric and substance use comorbidity among treatment-seeking opioid abusers. Arch Gen Psychiatry 1997;54:71–80.
4. Strain EC. Assessment and treatment of comorbid psychiatric disorders in opioid-dependent patients. Clin J Pain 2002;18:514–27.
5. Van de Brink W, Haasen C. Evidence-based treatment of opioid-dependent patients. Canada Journal of Psychiatry 2006;51:635–46.
6. Haug NA, Sorensen JL, Gruber VA, et al. Relapse prevention for opioid dependence. In: Mariatt GA, Donovan DM, editors. Relapse prevention: maintenance strategies in the treatment of addictive behaviors. 2nd edition. New York: Guilford Press; 2005. p. 151–78.
7. Mark TL, Woody GE, Juday T, et al. The economic costs of heroin addiction in the United States. Drug Alcohol Depend 2001;61:195–206.
8. Substance abuse and mental health services administration. Treatment episode data set 2007. Available at: www.oas.samhsa.gov/TEDS2k7highlights/TEDSHighl2k7Tbl4.htm. Accessed February 2, 2010.
9. Hayward MD, Schaich-Borg A, Pintar JE, et al. Differential involvement of endogenous opioids in sucrose consumption and food reinforcement. Pharmacol Biochem Behav 2006;85:601–11.
10. Shippenberg TS, Chefer VI, Thompson AC. Delta-opioid receptor antagonists prevent sensitization to the conditioned rewarding effects of morphine. Biol Psychiatry 2009;65(2):169–74.
11. Jaffe JH, Martin WR. Opioid analgesics and antagonists. In: Gilman AG, Rall TW, Nies AS, et al, editors. Goodman and Gilman's the pharmacological basis of therapeutics. 8th edition. New York: Pergamon Press; 1990. p. 485–521.
12. Marshall BE, Longnecker DE. General anesthetics. In: Gilman AG, Rall TW, Nies AS, et al, editors. Goodman and Gilman's the pharmacological basis of therapeutics. 8th edition. New York: Pergamon Press; 1990. p. 311–31.
13. Jaffe JH. Opiates: clinical aspects. In: Lowinson JH, Ruiz P, editors. Substance abuse a comprehensive textbook. 2nd edition. Baltimore (MD): Williams and Wilkins; 1992. p. 186–93.
14. Weinshenker D, Schroeder JP. There and back again: a tale of norepinephrine and drug addiction. Neuropsychopharmacology 2007;32:1433–51.
15. Wise RA. Addictive drugs and brain stimulation reward. Annu Rev Neurosci 1996; 19:340.
16. Cunha-Oliveira T, Rego AC. Cellular and molecular mechanisms involved in the neurotoxicity of opioid and psychostimulant drugs. Brain Res Rev 2008;58: 192–208.

17. Gold MS. The pharmacology of opioids. In: Graham AW, Schultz TK, editors. Principles of addiction medicine. 2nd edition. Maryland: American Society of Addiction Medicine, Inc; 1998. p. 131–6.
18. Nestler EJ. Basic neurobiology of opiate addiction. In: Stine SM, Kosten TR, editors. New treatements for opiate dependence. New York: Guilford Press; 1997. p. 286.
19. Strain EC, Stitzer ML. The treatment of opioid dependence. Baltimore (MD): Johns Hopkins Press; 2006. p. 275–94.
20. Strain EC. Pharmacology of buprenorphine. The treatment of opioid dependence. Baltimore (MD): Johns Hopkins Press; 2006. p. 213–29.
21. Helm S, Trescot AM, Colson J, et al. Opioid antagonists, partial agonists and agonists/antagonists: the role of office-based detoxification. Pain Physician 2008;11:225–35.
22. Saidak Z, Blake-Palmer K, Hay DL, et al. Differential activation of G-proteins by mu-opioid receptor agonists. Br J Pharmacol 2006;147:671–80.
23. American Psychiatric Association. Diagnostic and statistical manual of mental disorders. 4th edition. Washington, DC: American Psychiatric Association; 1994.
24. Schuckit MA, Segal DS. Opioid drug abuse and dependence. In: Kaspar DL, Braunwald E, editors. Harrison's principles of internal medicine. 16th edition. New York (NY): McGraw Hill; 2005. p. 2567–70.
25. O'Connor PG, Kosten TR. Management of opioid intoxication and withdrawal. In: Graham AW, Schultz TK, editors. Principles of addiction medicine. 2nd edition. Maryland: American Society of Addiction Medicine, Inc; 1998. p. 457–62.
26. Amato L, Davoli M. Methadone at tapered doses for the management of opioid withdrawal. Cochrane Database Syst Rev 2002;3:CD003409.
27. Gossop M. Medically supervised withdrawal as stand-alone treatment. In: Strain EC, Stitzer ML, editors. The treatment of opioid dependence. Baltimore (MD): Johns Hopkins Press; 2006. p. 346–62.
28. Nadelmann E, McNeely J. Doing methadone right. Public Interest 1996;123: 83–93.
29. O'Connor PG, Kosten TR. Rapid and ultrarapid opioid detoxification techniques. JAMA 1998;279:229–34.
30. Kienbaum P, Scherbaum N, Thürauf N, et al. Acute detoxification of opioid-addicted patients with naloxone during propofol or methohexital anesthesia: a comparison of withdrawal symptoms, neuroendocrine, metabolic, and cardiovascular patterns. Crit Care Med 2000;28:969–76.
31. Hamilton RJ, Olmedo RE, Shah S, et al. Complications of ultrarapid opioid detoxification with subcutaneous naltrexone pellets. Acad Emerg Med 2002; 9:63–8.
32. Collins ED, Kleber HD, Whittington RA, et al. Anesthesia-assisted vs buprenorphine- or clonidine-assisted heroin detoxification and naltrexone induction: a randomized trial. JAMA 2005;294:903–13.
33. Gowing L, Ali R, White J. Opioid antagonists under heavy sedation or anesthesia for opioid withdrawal. Cochrane Database Syst Rev 2006;1:CD002022.
34. Amato L, Minozzi S, Davoli M, et al. Psychosocial and pharmacological treatments versus pharmacological treatments for opioid detoxification. Cochrane Database Syst Rev 2004;4:CD005031.
35. Drug and treatment act of 2000. 21USC 2000. Available at: buprenorphine. samhsa.gov/data.html. Accessed February 10, 2010.
36. Physician waiver qualifications 2000. Available at: buprenorphine.samhsa.gov/ waiver_qualifications.html. Accessed February 10, 2010.

37. Zhang Z, Friedmann PD, Gerstein DR. Does retention mater? Treatment duration and improvement in drug use. Addiction 2003;98:673–8.
38. Mattick RP, Breen C, Kimber J, et al. Methadone maintenance therapy versus no opioid replacement therapy for opioid dependence. Cochrane Database Syst Rev 2003;2:CD002209.
39. Kakko J, Svanborg KD, Kreek MJ, et al. 1-year retention and social function after buprenorphine assisted relapse prevention treatment for heroin dependence in Sweden: a randomized, placebo-controlled trial. Lancet 2003;361:662–8.
40. Fiellin DA, O'Connor PG, Chawarski M, et al. Methadone maintenance in primary care: a randomized controlled trial. JAMA 2001;286:1724–31.
41. Faggiano F, Vigna-Taglianti F, Versino E, et al. Methadone maintenance at different dosages for opioid dependence. Cochrane Database Syst Rev 2003; 3:CD002208.
42. Gowing LR, Farrell M, Bornemann R, et al. Brief report: methadone treatment of injecting opioid users for prevention of HIV infection. J Gen Intern Med 2006; 21:193–9.
43. Pearson EC, Woosley RL. QT prolongation and torsades de pointes among methadone users: reports to the FDA spontaneous reporting system. Pharmacoepidemiol Drug Saf 2005;14:747.
44. Chugh SS, Socoteanu C, Reinier K, et al. A community-based evaluation of sudden death associated with therapeutic levels of methadone. Am J Med 2008;121:66–72.
45. Krantz MJ, Martin J, Stimmel B, et al. QTc interval screening in methadone treatment. Ann Intern Med 2009;150:387–93.
46. Mattick RP, Kimber J, Breen C, et al. Buprenorphine maintenance versus placebo or methadone maintenance for opioid dependence. Cochrane Database Syst Rev 2003;2:CD002207.
47. Barry DT, Moore BA, Pantalon MV, et al. Patient satisfaction with primary care office-based buprenorphine/naloxone treatment. J Gen Intern Med 2007;22:242–9.
48. National Institute for Health and Clinical Excellence (NICE). Methadone and buprenorphine for the management of opioid dependence. London: NICE; 2007.
49. Fischer G, Gombas W, Eder H, et al. Buprenorphine versus methadone maintenance for the treatment of opioid dependence. Addiction 1999;94:1337–44.
50. Schottenfeld RS, Pakes JR, Oliveto A, et al. Buprenorphine vs methadone maintenance treatment for concurrent opioid dependence and cocaine abuse. Arch gen psychiatry 1997;54:713–20.
51. Luty J, O'Gara C, Sessay M. Is methadone too dangerous for opiate addiction? BMJ 2005;331:1352–7.
52. Ling W, Compton P. Recent advances in the treatment of opiate addiction. Clin Neurosci Res 2005;6:161–7.
53. Jones ES, Moore BA, Sindelar JL, et al. Cost analysis of clinic and office-based treatment of opioid dependence: results with methadone and buprenorphine in clinically stable patients. Drug Alcohol Depend 2009;99:132.
54. Stein MD, Cioe P, Friedmann PD. Buprenorphine retention in primary care. J gen intern med 2005;20:1038–41.
55. Amato L, Minozzi S, Davoli M, et al. Psychosocial combined with agonist maintenance treatments versus agonist maintenance treatments alone for treatment of opioid dependence. Cochrane Database Syst Rev 2008;4:CD004147.
56. Christo G, Franey C. Drug users' spiritual beliefs, locus of control and the disease concepts in relation to Narcotics Anonymous attendance and six-month outcomes. Drug Alcohol Depend 1995;38:51–6.

57. Christo G, Sutton S. Anxiety and self-esteem as a function of abstinence time among recovering addicts attending Narcotics Anonymous. Br J Clin Psychol 1994;33:198–200.
58. Gossop M, Stewart D, Marsden J. Attendance at Narcotics Anonymous and Alcoholics Anonymous meetings, frequency of attendance and substance use outcomes after residential treatment for drug dependence: a 5-year follow-up study. Addiction 2008;103(1):119–25.

Prescription Drug Abuse: Epidemiology, Regulatory Issues, Chronic Pain Management with Narcotic Analgesics

Jeanne M. Manubay, MD[a,b,]*, Carrie Muchow, EdM[c], Maria A. Sullivan, MD, PhD[a,d]

KEYWORDS

- Opioids • Chronic pain • Prescription drug abuse
- Pain management

Although prescription drugs have been used effectively and appropriately to treat medical and psychiatric illnesses in most patients, rates of abuse have escalated at alarming rates in the past decade.[1] The increased availability of prescription drugs has contributed to a dramatic increase in nonmedical use and abuse of these medications.[2] Increased clinician awareness is essential in helping reduce prescription drug abuse while continuing to provide effective treatment.

In the last few decades, the treatment of chronic pain has expanded in the primary care setting.[3] Many primary care providers have had little specific training in pain medicine and addiction and are unsure about how to safely prescribe opioids.[4] In addition, the high prevalence of psychiatric comorbidity in those who misuse or abuse prescription drugs contributes to the complexity in treating pain.[5]

This work was supported by NIDA grant RO1 DA020448.

The authors have nothing to disclose.

[a] Division on Substance Abuse, New York State Psychiatric Institute, 1051 Riverside Drive, Unit 66, New York, NY 10032, USA

[b] Departments of Family Medicine and Psychiatry, Columbia University, 710 West 168th Street, New York, NY 10032, USA

[c] The Columbia University Buprenorphine Program, Department of Psychiatry, Columbia University, 710 West 168th Street, 12th Floor, New York, NY 10032, USA

[d] Department of Psychiatry, Columbia University, 710 West 168th Street, New York, NY 10032, USA

* Corresponding author. Division on Substance Abuse, New York State Psychiatric Institute, 1051 Riverside Drive, Unit 66, New York, NY 10032.

E-mail address: jmm2141@columbia.edu

Chronic pain conditions and prescription drug abuse are becoming important public health issues. Population-based studies reveal that more than 75 million Americans (about 25% of the entire population) have chronic or recurrent pain. Of these, 40% report the pain as having moderate to severe effect on their lives.[6] Chronic pain has placed an undue burden in lost productivity and is a frequent cause of disability, with an estimated cost to employees of more than $61 billion annually.[7] The prevalence of chronic pain conditions will only increase with the advancing age of our population.[8]

Navigating the complexity of treatment guidelines provided by the Federation of State Medical Boards, the US Drug Enforcement Agency (DEA), and other health organizations can be confusing and intimidating. The difficulties in measuring pain, fear of regulatory issues, and legal risks are additional barriers to providing appropriate pain management.

This article covers the epidemiology of prescription drug abuse, regulatory issues, and chronic pain management with narcotic analgesics. By understanding the scope of the problem, developing structured pain management plans, and being aware of aberrant behaviors, clinicians may feel more prepared and confident when dealing with acute and chronic pain.

EPIDEMIOLOGY

The most up-to-date and reliable sources on the epidemiology of prescription drug abuse include the National Survey on Drug Use and Health (NSDUH), the National Epidemiologic Survey on Alcohol and Related Conditions (NESARC), Monitoring the Future, and the Drug Abuse Warning Network (DAWN). These surveys collect different types of information that can give an accurate account of the trends of prescription drug abuse.

The NSDUH is an annual survey of the civilian noninstitutionalized population of the United States 12 years or older (N = 67,500), sponsored by Substance Abuse and Mental Health Services Administration (SAMHSA) Office of Applied Studies in the Department of Health and Human Services (DHHS).[9] The NSDUH has provided information on the incidence and prevalence of substance use in the population and the problems associated with use on an annual basis since 1999. In addition to describing the sociodemographic characteristics of users, patterns of use, treatment, perceptions of risk and availability, criminal behavior, and mental health, the NSDUH covers 4 broad classes of prescription psychotherapeutic drugs, including pain relievers, tranquilizers, stimulants, and sedatives. Nonmedical use is defined as the use of these medications without one's own prescription or simply for the experience of euphoria or other positive subjective drug effects. Neither does nonmedical use include the legitimate use of prescription drugs under a physician's direction nor does it include the use of over-the-counter (OTC) medications.

The most recent NSDUH statistics for 2008 reported an estimated 6.2 million (2.5%) persons 12 years or older using prescription-type psychotherapeutic drugs nonmedically in the past month.[9] Most nonmedical users (55.9%) obtained these drugs from a friend or relative for free (of which, 81.7% of these friends or relatives received drugs from 1 doctor).[9] About 18.0% of nonmedical users received these drugs from only 1 doctor.[9] Only 4.3% got pain relievers from a drug dealer or other strangers, and 0.4% bought them on the Internet.[9] For the first time, the largest number of past-year initiates (first-time users) of illicit drugs for persons 12 years or older were equal for marijuana use and nonmedical use of pain relievers (both 2.2 million).[9] While marijuana represented the illicit drug with the highest levels of past-year dependence or abuse at 4.2 million, pain relievers (1.7 million) are now the second most commonly abused illicit substances.[9]

New data on mental health were collected for 2008 NYSDUH reports, which revealed that adults with major depressive episodes (MDE) in the past year were more likely than those without MDE to depend on or abuse illicit drugs or alcohol (20.3% vs 7.8%).[9] Persons with serious mental illness (SMI) are defined as those 18 years or older who in the past year have had a *Diagnostic and Statistical Manual of Mental Disorders* (Fourth Edition) (DSM-IV)-based mental, behavioral, or emotional disorder (excluding developmental and substance use disorders) that meets diagnostic criteria, resulting in functional impairment in one or more major life activities. Among persons with SMI, the rate of past-year substance dependence or abuse was 25.3% (2.5 million) compared with 8.3% (17.9 million) for those without SMI.[9]

Compared with reports of past-month nonmedical use of pain relievers in 2002, there are increases among young adults aged 18 to 25 years (from 4.1%–4.6%) and adults 26 years or older (from 1.3%–1.6%) in 2007.[10] According to data from 2006 to 2008, among adults 50 years or older, an estimated 4.3 million (4.7%) had used an illicit drug in the past year. Thus, rates of nonmedical prescription drug use are currently increasing, particularly at both ends of the adult age spectrum. Indeed, among those who are 65 years and older, nonmedical use of prescription-type drugs is now more common than marijuana use (0.8% vs 0.4%).[11]

With regard to stimulants, educational activity seems to predict the likelihood of nonmedical use. Full-time college students aged 18 to 22 years were twice as likely to have used a combination of amphetamine and dextroamphetamine (Adderall) nonmedically in the past year compared with part-time students of the same age (6.4% vs 3.0%).[12] Those students who reported nonmedical use of Adderall were 8 times more likely than nonusers to be nonmedical users of prescription tranquilizers (24.5% vs 3.0%) and 5 times more likely to have concurrent nonmedical use of prescription pain relievers (44.9% vs 8.7%).[12]

NESARC was originally designed to study the magnitude of alcohol use disorders and their associated disabilities in the general population.[13] NESARC is sponsored by the US DHHS/National Institutes of Health/National Institute on Alcohol Abuse and Alcoholism. It is a longitudinal survey with its first wave of interviews fielded in 2001–2002 and the second wave in 2004–2005. The NESARC is a representative sample (43,093 respondents) of the noninstitutionalized US population 18 years and older.[13] Public use data are currently available for the first wave of data collection.

The NESARC collects data on alcohol consumption, alcohol abuse and dependence, alcohol treatment use, drug abuse and dependence, drug treatment use, family history of drug abuse, major depression, family history of major depression, and other psychiatric disorders.[13] Information on the nonmedical use of prescription opioids, sedatives, tranquilizers, and stimulants (which includes using without a prescription, using in greater amounts, using more often or longer than prescribed, or using for a reason other than a doctor's instruction) is also available.[13]

The lifetime prevalence of nonmedical prescription drug use in 2004–2005 was highest for opioids and stimulants (both 4.7%), followed by sedatives (4.1%) and tranquilizers (3.4%), and the lifetime prevalence of abuse or dependence for these drugs (nonmedical use) was highest for stimulants (2.0%), followed by opioids (1.4%), sedatives (1.1%), and tranquilizers (1.0%).[13] There were significant associations between nonmedical prescription drug use disorders and other substance use disorders as well as co-occurring DSM-IV Axes I and II psychiatric disorders, most notably alcohol abuse (odds ratio [OR], 11.4–16.1) and antisocial personality disorder (OR, 8.1–9.9).[13]

With regard to age categories, young adults aged 18 to 29 years had the highest rates of nonmedical use of opioids (7.4%) and tranquilizers (4.7%).[13] Those aged 30 to 44 years had higher rates of nonmedical use of stimulants (6.8%) and sedatives (5.1%).[13] The NESARC report also analyzes demographic and regional differences in nonmedical use and abuse of prescription drugs.[13] Men, especially in the western United States, had significantly higher rates than women, of nonmedical use of all categories of prescription drugs.[13] Native Americans also had the highest rates of prescription drug abuse in all categories, followed by Hispanics, Asians, and African Americans.[13] Compared with persons who were married and cohabitating, those who were never married, widowed, separated, or divorced had greater nonmedical use/abuse of opioids, sedatives, and tranquilizers.[13] Thus, risk factors for nonmedical use of prescription opioids include male gender, Native American or Hispanic ethnicity, and single status.

Monitoring the Future is an annual survey of high-school students in grades 8 to 12 and a smaller sample of previously surveyed high-school graduates that looks at the prevalence of drug and alcohol use.[14] In 2007, 48,025 students from 403 schools responded.[14] To determine nonmedical use of psychotropic medications, participants were asked about use "on your own, that is, without a doctor telling you to take them". Annual rates of nonmedical use of prescription opioids have more than doubled in high-school seniors in the last 15 years from 3.5% in 1991 to 9.2% in 2007.[14] The use of sedatives and tranquilizers has decreased from 11% in the mid-1970s to 6.2% in 2007.[14] Among the 12th graders, stimulant use has fluctuated through the years, from 20.3% in 1982 to 7.1% in 1992 and most recently to 7.5% in 2007.[14] When asked about availability of prescription medications, the percentage of 12th graders who reported that it was fairly easy or very easy to obtain drugs was 49.6% for stimulants, 41.7% for sedatives, 37.3% for opioids, and 23.6% for tranquilizers.[14]

DAWN is sponsored by SAMHSA and adds additional insight to the scope of the problem of nonmedical use and abuse of drugs. Data are collected from 355 nonfederal US hospitals that have 24-hour emergency departments (EDs).[15] DAWN reports track ED visits related to the recent use of prescription medications, OTC medications, dietary supplements, and alcohol.[15] In 2005, 1.5 million of the 108 million ED visits were associated with drug misuse or abuse, with most visits (55%) involving multiple drugs.[15] Of these visits, more than one-third involved the nonmedical use of prescription or OTC drugs.[15] In decreasing order, there were 204,711 visits related to anxiolytics, sedatives, and hypnotics; 196,225 visits for opioids; 61,023 visits for antidepressants; and 10,616 for stimulants (amphetamine, dextroamphetamine, methylphenidate, and caffeine).[15] In one DAWN report, there were an estimated 245,800 drug-related ED visits for patients diagnosed with co-occurring substance use and mental disorders in 2004.[16]

Although national surveys provide important information on the national burden of prescription drug misuse and abuse, there are limitations with regard to the methodology, measures, and sample populations targeted. More specific and recent trends can be captured from other sources, such as the Drug Evaluation Network System, which has valuable information on patients admitted to addiction treatment programs.[17] This system has detected increases in abuse of oxycodone hydrochloride (HCl) from 2002 to 2004.[17] Among the 27,816 subjects, 1425 (5%) reported ever using oxycodone HCl and a majority (87%) had used it more than thrice per week for at least 1 year.[17] The use of oxycodone HCl with at least one other opioid was reported by 92% of the users.[17] Abusers of oxycodone HCl were more likely to be White (89%), male (69%), younger (mean 32 ± 10 years), employed (51%), and to have used heroin compared with the rest of the group (all $P<.05$).[17]

Another trend is the use of Internet as a growing source of controlled prescription medications for nonmedical use.[18] The National Center on Addiction and Substance Abuse at Columbia University has reported an alarming increase in the number of Web sites selling controlled prescription drugs (ie, oxycodone HCl, acetaminophen/hydrocodone, diazepam, and methylphenidate) from 154 in 2004 to 187 in 2007.[19] Benzodiazepines are most frequently offered (sold on 79% of such sites), followed by opioids (in 64% of sites).[19] In another study, 735 sites offered opioids without a prescription.[18]

Online pharmacies have become a multibillion-dollar industry worldwide. In 2005, 32% of online customers surveyed reported having purchased medications or health care products on the Internet.[20] The availability of prescription drugs on the Internet increases the likelihood of unchecked medication interactions and side effects without reliable physician supervision. The use of cyberdoctor consultations to determine the need for prescriptions through online questionnaires raises concerns about whether such programs involve participation by actual physicians or if these are merely computer programs that help guide patients toward responses necessary to justify a prescription.[21] Few sites disclose the credentials of the doctors providing online services, and some state that physicians may not reside in the same country as the patient or the pharmacy.[22] Medications from these sites may also be expired, substandard, or counterfeit because Web sites are not required to provide information on where or when drugs are manufactured.[23]

The existence of Internet pharmacies allows individuals to bypass the traditional safeguards placed by the Food and Drug Administration (FDA), Congress, and health care providers, thereby placing consumers at risk.[24] The FDA, drug manufacturers, and professional organizations have been active in finding ways to reduce risk. The FDA Web site (www.fda.gov) provides useful information on how to spot and avoid health fraud and allows for reporting of suspicious sites. This system averages about 60,000 complaints per month.[25] The FDA Web site, www.fda.gov/oc/buyonline/others.html is also a reliable source for purchasing medications on the Internet, and www.fda.gov/ora/oasis/ora_oasis_ref.html lists international Web sites banned from offering prescription medications to people in the United States.

REGULATORY ISSUES

The epidemic of prescription drug abuse has gained enough public attention to warrant governmental hearings to address this issue. On July 26, 2006, there were testimonies before the SubCommittee on Criminal Justice, Drug Policy, and Human Resources, Committee On Government Reform, United States House of Representatives in a hearing titled Prescription Drug Abuse: What is Being Done to Address this New Drug Epidemic? Some key topics included what is being done at present as well as future strategies to combat drug abuse, including prescription drug monitoring programs, reducing malprescriptions, public education, eliminating Internet drug pharmacies, and the development of future drugs that are not only tamper resistant but also nonaddictive.

The DEA has been active in addressing the problems with prescription drug abuse. On October 27, 1970, The Comprehensive Drug Abuse Prevention and Control Act was passed by the Congress.[26] This Act was a "consolidation of numerous laws regulating the manufacturing and distribution of narcotics ... and chemicals used in the illicit production of controlled substances" and provided a "legal foundation of the government's fight against drugs and other substances."[26] The DEA's diversion control program is involved in overseeing and regulating the legal manufacture and distribution of controlled pharmaceuticals. The DEA recognizes that controlled pharmaceuticals can be diverted intentionally or unintentionally by doctors, pharmacists, dentists, nurses, veterinarians, and individual users. Such diversion cases include physicians selling prescriptions to drug dealers, pharmacists falsifying records to obtain and then sell pharmaceuticals, individuals who forge prescriptions, "doctor shoppers" who visit multiple doctors to obtain multiple prescriptions for the same ailment, and individuals using the Internet to sell controlled medications without requiring prescriptions.

Despite being criticized by the Congress in a 2005 House report for demonstrating a "lack of effort to address this problem," the DEA contends that it has significantly increased the amount of resources and manpower dedicated to the diversion of controlled pharmaceuticals by increasing the number of special agent work hours by 114% and the number of intelligence analysts by 234% from 2003 to 2005.[27,28] Other DEA efforts include an antidrug Web site for teenagers by the Demand Reduction Office, www.justthinktwice.com, which provides information on the consequences of drug use and trafficking as well as health, social, and legal consequences.[28] In addition, the Demand Reduction Office provides presentations to the public and school-aged children regarding the abuse of controlled prescriptions.[28]

Prescription drug monitoring programs were first developed in the early twentieth century to detect and prosecute diversion cases. With the collaboration of the American Society of Interventional Pain Physicians (ASIPP), the Congress passed and signed into law the National All Schedules Prescription Electronic Reporting (NASPER) Act on August 11, 2005 to establish or improve state-run prescription drug monitoring programs.[29] These statewide programs have served to track the flow of prescriptions of controlled medications. NASPER is housed within the Department of Health and Human Services and has been allocated $60 million through fiscal year 2010. Prescription monitoring programs (PMPs) first involve collecting data from physicians who prescribe medications and pharmacies that fill these prescriptions. Data collected can differ from state to state but often include the prescriber's name and DEA number, prescription date, the name and dose of the medication, the drug schedule code, and the patient's name and date of birth. Data are stored and centrally processed, usually by a state government agency, and each state has varying rules as to how these data are made available to authorized persons and agencies. Physicians, pharmacists, and law enforcement officials may acquire information with the goal toward preventing prescription drug abuse.

The development of these programs has been slow, and funding has not been guaranteed. In 2007, 38 states had established PMPs. California developed the triplicate prescription form in the 1940s, which became a gold standard for data collection. This system was replaced in California with an electronic prescription system in 1998, which many states have adopted. Because many programs are new, their effectiveness is difficult to determine. Recent data suggest that the proactive use of PMP's results in lower sales of prescription medications.[30] Another study suggests that although these programs have helped shift prescription practice, the rates of prescription drug abuse have not been reduced.[31]

At the state level, state laws govern prescription drug prescribing and dispensing of licensed clinicians. State Medical Licensure Boards respond to complaints but do not actively seek out problematic prescribing practices.

Public education of authorities, physicians, pharmacists, and patients can help to inform about the problems of drug abuse as well as provide warning signs and strategies to combat abuse. Organizations such as Partnership for a Drug-Free America, state and local agencies, and medical and pharmaceutical societies have made efforts to educate the public. Similarly, at the federal level, organizations such as the Office of the National Drug Control Policy, the National Institute on Drug Abuse to Prevent and Treat Prescription Drug Abuse, the Department of Health and Human Services, and the SAMHSA have also helped to inform and warn of the epidemic of prescription drug abuse.

Research efforts to understand factors that influence vulnerability to addiction, as well as factors that predispose or protect against opioid abuse, are being funded through programs such as the National Institute on Drug Abuse (NIDA).[32] The influence of genetic factors on vulnerability to addiction in those exposed to pain medication are also of great interest to NIDA.

The Federal Food, Drug, and Cosmetic Act mandates that the FDA ensure that all new drugs are safe and effective.[33] The FDA must assess a drug's potential for abuse and misuse based on drug chemistry, pharmacology clinical manifestations, as well as the potential for public health risks after introducing it to the general population.[33] Once the abuse potential is determined, a drug is assigned to 1 of 5 schedules, depending on the abuse potential and medical use, as defined by the Controlled Substances Act. The FDA also seeks expert advice from nonagency experts on the medical use of opioid analgesics. In September 2003, the FDA met with the DEA officials, pain and addiction specialists, to discuss the medical use of opioid analgesics, appropriate drug development plans to support approval of opioid analgesics, and strategies to communicate and manage risks associated with opioid analgesics, especially the risks of abuse of these drugs. The FDA is committed to protecting the public health by assuring that safe and effective products reach the market in a timely manner and monitoring products for continued safety after they become available. By working with federal agencies, professional societies, industry, and patient advocacy groups, information can be shared to minimize risk. The FDA also participates in risk minimization action plans, which are safety programs targeted to reduce product risks by using interventions such as restrictions on prescribing, dispensing, or using.

Another effort to minimize prescription drug abuse is the development of drugs that are tamper resistant and minimize the potential for abuse or diversion. The epidemic of oxycodone HCl (OxyContin) abuse highlights the difficulties in creating tamper-resistant formulations. Although initially intended to be slowly released over 12 hours, drug abusers were able to quickly learn how to disable physically or manually the controlled-release mechanism and extract oxycodone, a potent opioid, in order to experience a powerful and immediate high when ingested, snorted, or injected, which increased its addiction potential. One way to prevent tampering is to take advantage of pharmaceutical technology, such as using tamper-resistant capsules that are resistant to degradation by the usual methods that drug users use to destroy the extended-release mechanisms, such as chewing or crushing. Another approach is by combining an opioid agonist and antagonist (eg, oxycodone/naltrexone [Oxytrex]). Buprenorphine-naloxone developed for the treatment of opioid addiction has also proved to be effective as a pain medication with minimum abuse potential. Continued efforts at the development of formulations that are effective yet tamper resistant are now encouraged by the synthetic drug control strategy of the Office of the National Drug Control Policy with the goal of reducing diversion and abuse.[34]

Because physicians are the source of prescription drugs, we must be prudent to educate and provide training at all levels to ensure that physicians are aware of appropriate pain management and warning signs of drug abuse. Past surveys have indicated that less than 40% of physicians have received any training during medical school in identifying prescription drug use and addiction or drug diversion. In 2004, the rates of prescribing OxyContin and oxycodone had increased to 556% since 1997 in the United States. Without adequate knowledge of the long-term safety and appropriate use of opioids, physicians may unknowingly contribute to prescription drug abuse. Physicians must also educate patients about the storage of prescription medications and warn about the risks of sharing these medications with family and friends.

CHRONIC PAIN MANAGEMENT WITH NARCOTIC ANALGESICS

The use of narcotic analgesics for chronic pain management should be based on the need for long-term chronic opioid therapy (COT) after a comprehensive evaluation, a trial of nonnarcotic medications, and an awareness of potential risks for opioid abuse, dependence, and diversion. Once the need for long-term opioid treatment of pain management has been determined, physicians should consider a 10-step approach (**Table 1**).[35] This process begins with a thorough medical evaluation including diagnostic studies (ie, radiographs, magnetic resonance imaging) to establish medical diagnoses and medical necessity for COT, but also considers whether treatment is beneficial (ie, risk-benefit ratio), and addresses treatment strategies (eg, informed consent and written agreements, dose initiation, adjustment, and stabilization, adherence monitoring). Treatment goals should be defined, including outcome measures and decisions. Physicians must consider if COT is necessary, and the knowledge of patient selection and risk stratification, including the use of opioids in high-risk patients, requires the careful implementation of essential monitoring tools, such as assessment of aberrant drug-related behaviors, use of informed consent forms, controlled substance agreements, and risk assessment tools.

The definition of chronic pain is "pain that persists beyond normal tissue healing time, which is assumed to be three months."[36] The 3-step World Health Organization ladder for cancer pain has been widely used and adapted for the treatment of chronic noncancer pain (**Fig. 1**).[37] Step 1 recommends the use of nonopioid medication, with or without an adjuvant medication, if necessary. Adjuvant medications include antidepressants, anticonvulsants, and corticosteroids and are used to enhance analgesic effect, to treat concurrent symptoms that may exacerbate pain, and to provide an independent analgesic effect. If pain increases, step 2 recommends taking an opioid medication that is used for mild to moderate pain along with a nonopioid medication and an adjuvant medication, if necessary. If pain increases further, step 3 recommends taking an opioid medication for moderate to severe pain along with nonopioid medication and an adjuvant medication, if necessary.

The American Pain Society, in collaboration with the American Academy of Pain Medicine, recently published evidence-based guidelines on the use of COT for chronic noncancer pain.[38] The key clinical messages have been summarized[39] and will be discussed in this section.

RISK ASSESSMENT AND STRATIFICATION

With regard to patient selection and stratification, a physician should routinely incorporate measures to assess risk for opioid abuse. All evaluations must start with a comprehensive physical examination; the medical history should also explore psychosocial factors and family history, which can help to determine risk stratification. A personal or family history of alcohol or drug abuse is the factor most strongly predictive of opioid abuse, misuse, or aberrant drug-related behavior.[3,40] Other predictors include a younger age and the presence of psychiatric conditions.[3,41] Some tools that may be useful to quantify risk in a clinical setting include the Screener and Opioid

Table 1
The 10-step process: an algorithmic approach for long-term opioid therapy in chronic pain

Step 1	Comprehensive initial evaluation
Step 2	Establish diagnosis Radiographs, MRI, CT, neurophysiological studies Psychological evaluation Precision diagnostic interventions
Step 3	Establish medical necessity (lack of progress or as supplemental therapy) Physical diagnosis Therapeutic interventional pain management Physical modalities Behavior therapy
Step 4	Assess risk-benefit ratio Treatment is beneficial
Step 5	Establish treatment goals
Step 6	Obtain informed consent and agreement
Step 7	Initial dose adjustment phase (up to 8–12 wk) Start low dose Use opioids, NSAIDS, and adjuvants Discontinue due to Lack of analgesia Side effects Lack of functional improvement
Step 8	Stable phase (stable, moderate doses) Monthly refills Assess for 4 A's Analgesia Activity Aberrant behavior Adverse effect Manage side effects
Step 9	Adherence monitoring PMPs Random drug screens Pill counts
Step 10	Outcomes Success, continue Stable doses Analgesia, activity No abuse, side effects Failed, discontinue if Dose escalation No analgesia No activity Abuse Side effects Noncompliance

Abbreviations: CT, computed tomography; MRI, magnetic resonance imaging; NSAIDs, nonsteroidal antiinflammatory drugs.
From Trescot AM, Boswell MV, Atluri SL, et al. Opioid guidelines in the management of chronic non-cancer pain. Pain Phys 2006;9:26; with permission.

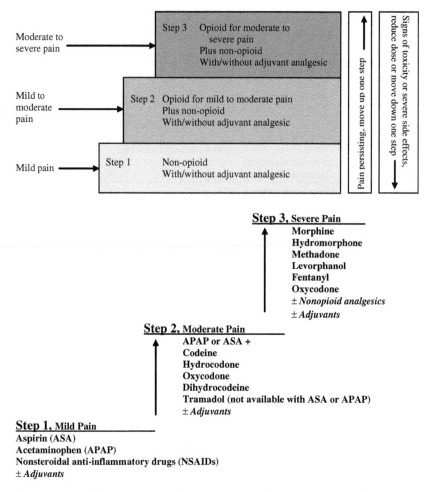

"Adjuvants" refers either to medications that are coadministered to manage an adverse effect of an opioid, or to so-called adjuvant analgesics that are added to enhance analgesia.

Fig. 1. WHO pain ladder. (*Adapted from* World Health Organization. Cancer pain relief and palliative care. Geneva: WHO; 1996; with permission.)

Assessment for Patients with Pain (SOAPP) Version 1, the revised SOAPP, the Opioid Risk Tool, and the Diagnosis, Intractability, Risk, Efficacy Tool.

Only when potential benefits outweigh risks, and when other nonopioid options have been maximized, should OT be considered. A thorough discussion with patients of common opioid side effects (ie, constipation, nausea, sedation), other risks (ie, abuse, addiction, overdose), and known potential long-term risks (ie, hyperalgesia, endocrinologic or sexual dysfunction) is essential when considering COT. Once it is determined that opioid therapy should be initiated, clinicians should administer informed consent and have the document signed by the patient (**Fig. 2**). Patients should be told about the need to keep controlled substances in a safe and locked location, if possible, to prevent diversion or easy access from friends or other family members. A controlled substance agreement is helpful to address expectations and goals and describe clinical follow-up and monitoring, rules for lost prescriptions and requests for early refills, and consequences of noncompliance, such as tapering or discontinuing COT when therapeutic goals are not met, side effects become intolerable, or serious aberrant behaviors have been identified (**Fig. 3**).

Screening for addiction should always be done at the start of treatment. Stratifying patients into risk categories for addiction liability will make it easier for a clinician to determine individualized treatment strategies, including the need for outside referrals.[42] It is advisable for clinicians to use universal precautions in order to triage individuals to different categories (low, medium, and high risk) in terms of addiction liability.[43]

Low-risk patients with chronic noncancer pain have no history of substance abuse and lack any major psychiatric comorbidity. There are no indications of aberrant behaviors or any warning signs that they may abuse medications in such patients. These individuals can be managed in a primary care setting.

Medium-risk patients may have a prior history of substance abuse or may have psychiatric comorbidity. These individuals can be managed in a primary care setting, particularly with consultation from a specialist (ie, an addiction specialist or a psychiatrist).

High-risk patients are those with active addictive disorders. These individuals are at an increased risk for aberrant behaviors and should be referred to a tertiary care clinic that specializes in pain management.

Another measure to help guide clinicians with their therapeutic decisions is the Pain Assessment and Documentation Tool (PADT).[44] This tool incorporates an assessment of the 4 A's: analgesia, activity, adverse effects, and aberrant behavior. It is important to identify aberrant behaviors because they may signal potential misuse of opioids. Certain aberrant behaviors have been demonstrated to reliably indicate a substance abuse disorder.[45,46] Such behaviors range from failing to comply with a prescribed regimen to clearly illegal behaviors, including selling prescription drugs, forging prescriptions, stealing drugs, injecting oral formulations, obtaining prescription drugs from nonmedical sources, concurrently abusing alcohol or other illicit drugs, escalating doses on multiple occasions or otherwise failing to comply with the prescribed regimen despite warnings, losing prescribed medications on multiple occasions, repeatedly seeking prescriptions from other clinicians or from emergency rooms without informing the original prescribing physician, and showing evidence of deterioration in the ability to function (at work, in the family, or socially), which seems to be related to drug use. The occurrence of any of these behaviors should warrant evaluation and more rigorous monitoring.

The presence of multiple aberrant behaviors or the recurrence of any of these behaviors may suggest the need for consultation with pain management physicians or addiction specialists. Clinicians should also consider temporary or permanent tapering of opioid doses and possibly discontinuation if more serious behaviors are evident (ie, diversion or intravenous use of oral formulations). Psychiatric referrals or psychological support with individual counseling (ie, cognitive behavioral therapy) may be helpful for some individuals, which highlights the need to screen for depression, anxiety, and other psychiatric disorders at the beginning of COT. For patients identified with an opioid addiction, structured opioid agonist therapy with buprenorphine or methadone at a licensed program may be beneficial to help treat pain and addiction.

For patients with low to medium risk for addiction liability, opioids should be started in a short-term therapeutic trial. In individuals who are opioid naive and in the elderly opioids should be started at low doses and titrated slowly. Short-acting opioids may

Consent for Chronic Opioid Therapy

A consent form from the **American Academy of Pain Medicine**

Dr. _____ is prescribing opioid medicine sometimes called narcotic analgesics, to me
for a diagnosis of _____.

This decision was made because my condition is serious or other treatments have not helped my pain.

I am aware that the use of such medicine has certain risks associated with it, including but not limited to:
sleepiness or drowsiness, constipation, nausea, itching, vomiting, dizziness, allergic reaction, slowing of
breathing rate, slowing of reflexes or reaction time, physical dependence, tolerance to analgesia, addiction
and possibly that the medicine will not provide complete pain relief.

I am aware about the possible risks and benefits of other types of treatments that do not involve the use of
opioids. The other treatments discussed included:
_____
_____
_____

I will tell my doctor about all other medicines and treatments that I am receiving.

I will not be involved in any activity that may be dangerous to me or someone else if I feel drowsy or am
not thinking clearly. I am aware that even if I do not notice it, my reflexes and reaction time might still be
slowed. Such activities include, but are not limited to: using heavy equipment or a motor vehicle, working
in unprotected heights or being responsible for another individual who is unable to care for himself or
herself.

I am aware that certain other medicines such as nalbuphine (Nubain™), pentazocine (Talwin™),
buprenorphine (Buprenex™), and butorphanol (Stadol™), may reverse the action of the medicine I am using
for pain control. Taking any of these other medicines while I am taking my pain medicines can cause
symptoms like a bad flu, called a withdrawal syndrome. I agree not to take any of these medicines and to
tell any other doctors that I am taking an opioid as my pain medicine and cannot take any of the medicines
listed above.

I am aware that addiction is defined as the use of a medicine even if it causes harm, having cravings for a
drug, feeling the need to use a drug and a decreased quality of life. I am aware that the chance of becoming
addicted to my pain medicines is very low. I am aware that the development of addiction has been reported
rarely in medical journals and is much more common in a person who has a family or personal history of
addiction. I agree to tell my doctor my complete and honest personal drug history and that of my family to
the best of my knowledge.

I understand that physical dependence is a normal, expected result of using these medicines for a long time.
I understand that physical dependence is not the same as addiction. I am aware physical dependence means
that if my pain medicine use is markedly decreased, stopped or reversed by some of the agents mentioned
above, I will experience withdrawal syndrome. This means I may have any or all of the following: runny
nose, yawning, large pupils, goose bumps, abdominal pain and cramping, diarrhea, irritability, aches
throughout my body and a flu-like feeling. I am aware that opioid withdrawal is uncomfortable but not life
threatening.

I am aware that tolerance to analgesia means that I may require more medicine to get the same amount of
pain relief. I am aware that tolerance to analgesia does not seem to be a big problem for most patients with
chronic pain, however, it has been seen and may occur to me. If it occurs, increasing doses may not always
help and may cause unacceptable side effects. Tolerance or failure to respond well to opioids may cause
my doctor to choose another form of treatment.

(**Males only**) I am aware that chronic opioid use has been associated with low testosterone levels in males.
This may affect my mood, stamina, sexual desire and physical and sexual performance. I understand that
my doctor may check my blood to see if my testosterone level is normal.

Fig. 2. Informed consent for COT. (Copyright © 1999 American Academy of Pain Medicine.
Reproduced with permission.)

(**Females only**) If I plan to become pregnant or believe that I have become pregnant while taking this pain medicine, I will immediately call my obstetric doctor and this office to inform them. I am aware that, should I carry a baby to delivery while taking these medicines, the baby will be physically dependent upon opioids. I am aware that the use of opioids is not generally associated with a risk of birth defects. However, birth defects can occur whether or not the mother is on medicines and there is always the possibility that my child will have a birth defect while I am taking an opioid.

I have read this form or have it read to me. I understand all of it. I have had a chance to have all of my questions regarding this treatment answered to my satisfaction. By signing this form, voluntarily, I give my consent for the treatment of my pain with opioid pain medicines.

Patient signature _____ Date _____

Witness to above _____

Approved by the AAPM Executive Committee on January 14, 1999

Fig. 2. (*continued*)

be safer because of a shorter half-life and a lower risk of unintentional overdose. However, the use of long-acting opioids may provide more consistent pain relief and better adherence. Although long-acting opioids were originally thought to have a lower potential for abuse and addiction, studies have proved otherwise.[47] For most opioids, a dosing schedule of 2 to 4 times daily is recommended to provide continuous coverage for pain relief. Additional, but limited, amounts of breakthrough doses should also be available, which may help patients gain a greater sense of control over pain. After initiation of an opioid, if the pain relief is inadequate, the dose can be increased after 3 days; subsequent dose titrations can be made in 24-hour periods. Because there is an absence of a ceiling effect with full-agonist opioids, doses can be increased until a desired analgesic effect is reached or until side effects are intolerable.

Caution should be used when prescribing methadone. There has been an increase in methadone-associated deaths that may be related to cardiac arrhythmias or unintentional overdoses because of its very long and variable half-life.[48] The half-life of methadone ranges from 15 to 60 hours, which means it could take up to 12 days to reach a steady state level. A safe starting dose is 2.5 mg every 8 hours, with dose increases only once per week. For opioid-tolerant individuals transitioning from high doses of other opioids, the starting methadone doses should not exceed 30 to 40 mg/d.

Common side effects of opioids should also be addressed. Constipation may be treated with stool softeners or other laxatives. For opioid-induced constipation, stimulant laxatives are recommended. Nausea and vomiting, which may occur during initiation of opioid therapy, can be treated by a variety of antiemetics. Sedation may require a reduction in dose. Routine testing for hormonal deficiencies should only be done for symptoms of decreased libido, sexual dysfunction, or fatigue. There is some evidence that opioid antagonist therapy may reduce glycemic control,[49,50] in part through a delayed insulin response resulting from opioid-induced intestinal slowing,[51,52] and monitoring of glucose levels may be warranted for patients demonstrating weight gain or at risk for diabetes mellitus.

Monitoring should be done frequently at the start of treatment to assess pain relief, adverse effects, and for dose adjustments. For patients who are elderly, have a history of substance abuse, or in whom mental acuity is particularly important for occupational purposes, visits should also be more frequent. The use of monitoring tools, such as the PADT,[44] or the Chronic Opioid Misuse Measure[53] can help with therapeutic decisions while assessing for risk. Urine drug testing is recommended,

We are committed to doing all we can to treat your chronic pain condition. In some cases, controlled substances are used as a therapeutic option in the management of chronic pain and related anxiety and depression, which is strictly regulated by both state and federal agencies. This agreement is a tool to protect both you and the physician by establishing guidelines, within the laws, for proper controlled substance use. The words "we" and "our" refer to the facility and the words "I", "you", "your", "me", or "my" refer to you, the patient.

1.   i. I understand that chronic opioid therapy has been associated with not only addiction and abuse, but also multiple medical problems including the suppression of endocrine function resulting in low hormonal levels in men and women which may affect mood, stamina, sexual desire, and physical and sexual performance.

ii. For female patients, if I plan to become pregnant or believe that I have become pregnant while taking this medication, I am aware that, should I carry the baby to delivery while taking these medications; the baby will be physically dependent upon opioids. I will immediately call my obstetrician and this office to inform them of my pregnancy. I am also aware that opioids may cause a birth defect, even though it is extremely rare.

iii. I have been informed that long-term and/or high doses of pain medications may also cause increased levels of pain known as opioid induced hyperalgesia (pain medicine causing more pain) where simple touch will be predicted as pain and pain gradually increases in intensity and also the location with hurting all over the body. I understand that opioid-induced hyperalgesia is a normal, expected result of using these medicines for a long period of time. This is only treated with addition of non-steroidal anti-inflammatory drugs such as Advil, Ibuprofen, etc., or by reducing or stopping opioids.

iv. I understand that physical dependence is not the same as addiction. I am aware physical dependence means that if my pain medicine use is markedly decreased, stopped, or reversed by some of the agents mentioned above, I will experience a withdrawal syndrome. This means I may have any or all of the following: runny nose, yawning, large pupils, goose bumps, abdominal pain and cramping, diarrhea, irritability, aches throughout my body and a flu-like feeling. I am aware that opioid withdrawal is uncomfortable, but not life threatening.

v. I am aware that tolerance to analgesia means that I may require more medicine to get the same amount of pain relief. I am aware that tolerance to analgesia does not seem to be a big problem for most patients chronic pain; however, it has been seen and may occur to me. If it occurs, increasing doses may not always help and may cause unacceptable side effects. Tolerance or failure to respond well to opioids may cause my doctor to choose another form of treatment, reduce the dose, or stop it.

2.   i. All controlled substances must come from the physician whose signature appears below or during his/her absence, by the covering physician, unless specific authorization is obtained for an exception.

ii. I understand that I must tell the physician whose signature appears below or during his/her absence, the covering physician, all drugs that I am taking, have purchased, or have obtained, even over-the-counter medications. Failure to do so may result in drug interactions or overdoses that could result in harm to me, including death.

iii. I will not seek prescriptions for controlled substances from any other physician, health care provider, or dentist. I understand it is unlawful to be prescribed the same controlled medication by more than one physician at a time without each physician's knowledge.

iv. I also understand that it is unlawful to obtain or to attempt to obtain a prescription for a controlled substance by knowingly misrepresenting facts to a physician or his/her staff or knowingly withholding facts from a physician or his/her staff (including failure to inform the physician or his/her staff of all controlled substances that I have been prescribed).

Fig. 3. A sample of controlled substance agreement. (*From* Trescot AM, Helm S, Hansen H, et al. Opioids in the management of chronic non-cancer pain: an update of American Society of the Interventional Pain Physicians' (ASIPP) guidelines. Pain Phys 2008;11:S48–9; with permission.)

especially in high-risk patients, and can determine the presence or absence of opioids prescribed and can detect the presence of other illicit drugs. If routine monitoring is too costly, random testing can still be beneficial. Pill counts can help determine if patients are compliant with treatment recommendations. Discussions with family members and caretakers may also provide valuable information about a patient's level of functioning. PMPs vary by state, but may be helpful in identifying patients who may be seeking controlled substances from multiple doctors and who may be abusing prescription drugs.

When dose escalations reach upper limits, physicians should inquire about analgesic effect, function, quality of life, adverse side effects, and aberrant drug behaviors. If pain relief is not optimal at the highest dose of opioid prescribed, physicians must first evaluate any changes in health status. Opioid rotation may then be considered, which refers to the substitution of one opioid for another, when pain relief is

3. All controlled substances must be obtained at the same pharmacy where possible. Should the need arise to change pharmacies, our office must be informed. The pharmacy that you have selected is: _____Phone:_____

4. i. You may not share, sell, or otherwise permit others, including your spouse or family members, to have access to any controlled substances that you have been prescribed.

    ii. Early refills will not be given. Renewals are based upon keeping scheduled appointments. Please do not make excessive phone calls for prescriptions or early refills and do not phone for refills after hours or on weekends.

5. Unannounced pill counts, random urine or serum, or planned drug screening may be requested from you and your cooperation is required. Presence of unauthorized substances in urine or serum toxicology screens may result in your discharge from the facility and its physicians and staff.

6. I will not consume excessive amounts of alcohol in conjunction with controlled substances. I will not use, purchase, or otherwise obtain any other legal drugs except as specifically authorized by the physician whose signature appears below or during his/her absence, by the covering physician, as set forth in Section 2 above. I will not use, purchase, or otherwise obtain any illegal drugs, including marijuana, cocaine, etc. I understand that driving while under the influence of any substance, including a prescribed controlled substance or any combination of substances (e.g., alcohol and prescription drugs), which impairs my driving ability, may result in DUI charges.

7. Medications or written prescriptions may not be replaced if they are lost, stolen, get wet, are destroyed, left on an airplane, etc. If your medication has been stolen, it will not be replaced unless explicit proof is provided with direct evidence from authorities. A report narrating what you told the authorities is not enough.

8. In the event you are arrested or incarcerated related to legal or illegal drugs (including alcohol), refills on controlled substances will not be given.

9. I understand that failure to adhere to these policies may result in cessation of therapy with controlled substances prescribed by this physician and other physicians at the facility and that law enforcement officials may be contacted.

10. I also understand that the prescribing physician has permission to discuss all diagnostic and treatment details, including medications, with dispensing pharmacists, other professionals who provide your health care or appropriate drug and law enforcement agencies for the purpose of maintaining accountability.

11. I affirm that I have full right and power to sign and to be bound by this agreement, that I have read it, and understand and accept all of its terms. A copy of this document has been given to me.

_____
Patient's full name

_____   _____
Patient's signature   Date

_____   _____
Physician's signature   Date

Fig. 3. (continued)

inadequate or when side effects become intolerable. It is recommended to switch with a moderate reduction in the calculated equianalgesic dose.[54]

Discontinuation of COT should be considered when patients are not meeting therapeutic goals, adverse effects are intolerable, or if serious or repeated aberrant behaviors have been identified. More complicated cases in terms of medical or psychiatric comorbidity may be managed better in a detoxification or rehabilitation center, and cases in which addiction is apparent are best referred to addiction specialists.

When tapering opioids, physicians can reduce the dose slowly, with a 10% dose reduction per week, or more rapidly, with a 25% to 50% dose reduction every few days, depending on patient comfort and length of time the patient has been on COT. In general, doses can be tapered rapidly until the daily doses of morphine (or equivalent) have reached 60 to 80 mg/d, when patients may experience more withdrawal symptoms, which may include pain hypersensitivity. Nonopioid medications should be used during this taper while psychiatric and substance abuse issues are addressed.

There is no strong evidence that patients maintained on stable doses of opioid without impairment should be restricted from driving.[55] However, those individuals in certain professions (ie, bus drivers, pilots) may be subject to strict regulations regarding the use of opioids. All patients who initiate opioid therapy, or are told to increase their dose, should be warned about the potential for sedation and to use caution with driving or other dangerous work. Patients should also be educated about the risks of taking other drugs or alcohol while on opioids. Any suspicion or demonstration of any dangerous behaviors (ie, driving when somnolent, incoordination) should be reported to the appropriate authorities.

The requirement for only a single prescribing physician or facility to administer opioids should be delineated in a treatment agreement. When all care can be established at one medical office, referrals can be better coordinated and problematic behaviors can be identified. The presence of a patient-centered primary care medical home can facilitate the multidimensional care that a patient needs.[56]

The use of COT can be safe and effective when physicians possess the clinical skills and knowledge to address all the facets of appropriate opioid management. With thorough ongoing clinical assessments and the use of screening tools and treatment agreements physicians can better determine if opioid therapy is beneficial or if consultations are warranted. Ongoing evaluations can guide any change in treatment and improve communication between the physician and patient. When goals have not been met or aberrant behaviors have been identified treatment agreements can delineate courses of action. By understanding the assessment and management of risk, a physician will also provide more effective treatment of chronic pain.

SUMMARY

The epidemic of prescription drug abuse has reached a level at which national attention has forced physicians to reevaluate the need to provide appropriate care to patients while understanding the potential risks of diversion and abuse of prescription drugs. The statistics and strategies in this article have highlighted the importance of educating ourselves and our patients, and being aware of the increased rates of prescription drug abuse, particularly among young adults, full-time college students, the elderly, and in those with SMI.

The development of prescription drug monitoring programs and NASPER are steps toward prevention and better detection of prescription drug abuse. The FDA, DEA, Office of the National Drug Control Policy, NIDA, SAMHSA, and organizations such as Partnership for a Drug-Free America have all made serious efforts to address this epidemic. With the collaboration of pain societies (ie, ASIPP), the Congress has made targeted and well-informed attempts to join the crusade against prescription drug abuse by signing laws, such as NASPER, and holding hearings to better understand the issues and formulate guidelines to help physicians prescribe opioids safely and effectively. Pharmaceutical companies are also developing innovative tamper-resistant formulations. Better education in medical schools of pain management and substance abuse is necessary. It is also imperative that public service organizations continue to educate parents and the public about warning signs of abuse, and preventative tips, such as not sharing medications with family and friends or keeping controlled substances in a safe, and preferably locked, location.

Physicians should also inform their patients of the risks of prescription drugs. Only after a careful and thorough assessment of a patient's medical conditions, with confirmatory diagnostic information and assessment of risk-benefit ratio, should physicians consider starting opioid therapy. All nonopioid medications or therapies should first be maximized and contributing psychological issues addressed. Informed consent and a treatment agreement should be discussed and signed before the start of treatment.

Risk assessment tools can help triage patients to determine the intensity and frequency of visits, and need for consultation. Monitoring tools and urine drug testing are also helpful when administering COT. An evaluation of the 4 A's at all visits is essential to evaluate success or to determine a need for change in management, such as dose escalation or discontinuation. If treatment agreements are violated in cases in which serious or repeated aberrant behaviors have been detected, discontinuation or transfer of care are more easily addressed when rules have been delineated. With the knowledge of the appropriate use of opioids and the risks involved an organized approach toward assessing and managing pain can facilitate the development of individualized treatment plans that maximize patient comfort, satisfaction, and safety. It is our duty as physicians to provide the best quality care to our patients, and well-informed opioid management should serve to reduce the epidemic of prescription drug abuse.

REFERENCES

1. Substance Abuse and Mental Health Services Administration. Results from the 2006 survey on drug use and health: national findings. DHHS publication SMA 07-4293. Rockville (MD): Office of Applied Studies; 2007.
2. McCabe SE, Teter CJ, Boyd CJ. Medical use, illicit use, and diversion of abusable prescription drugs. J Am Coll Health 2006;54:269–78.
3. Reid MC, Engles-Horton LL, Weber MB, et al. Use of opioid medications for chronic noncancer pain syndromes in primary care. J Gen Intern Med 2002;17:173–9.
4. Savage SR, Joranson DE, Covington EC, et al. Definitions related to the medical use of opioids: evolution towards universal agreement. J Pain Symptom Manage 2003;26:655–67.
5. Chelminski PR, Ives TJ, Felix KM, et al. A primary care, multi-disciplinary disease management program for opioid-treated patients with chronic non-cancer pain and a high burden of psychiatric comorbidity. BMC Health Serv Res 2005;5:1–13.
6. National Center for Health Statistics. Health, United States, 2006 with chartbook on trends in the health of Americans. Hyattsville (MD): NCHS; 2006. p. 68–71.
7. Stewart WF, Ricci JA, Chee E, et al. Lost productive time and cost due to common pain conditions in the US workforce. JAMA 2003;290:2443–54.
8. Clark JD. Chronic pain prevalence and analgesic prescribing in a general medical population. J Pain Symptom Manage 2002;23:131–7.
9. Substance Abuse and Mental Health Services Administration. Results from the 2008 National Survey on Drug Use and Health: national findings. NSDUH Series H-36, HHS Publication No. SMA 09–4434. Rockville (MD): Office of Applied Studies; 2009.
10. SAMHSA. The NSDUH report: trends in nonmedical use of prescription pain relievers: 2002 to 2007. Rockville (MD): Office of Applied Studies; 2009.
11. SAMHSA. The NSDUH report: illicit drug use among older adults. Rockville (MD): Office of Applied Studies; 2009.
12. SAMHSA. The NSDUH report: nonmedical use of Adderall among full-time college students. Rockville (MD): Office of Applied Studies; 2009.
13. Huang B, Dawson DA, Stinson FS, et al. Prevalence, correlates, and comorbidity of nonmedical prescription drug use and drug use disorders in the United States: results of the national epidemiologic survey on alcohol and related conditions. J Clin Psychiatry 2006;67:1062–73.

14. Johnston LD, O'Malley PM, Bachman JG, et al. Monitoring the future: national results on adolescent drug use: overview of key findings 2005. NIH publication 06-5882. Bethesda (MD): National Institute on Drug Abuse; 2006.
15. Substance Abuse and Mental Health Services Administration. Drug abuse warning network, 2005: national estimates of drug-related emergency department visits. DHHS publication (SMA) 07–4256. Rockville (MD): Office of Applied Studies; 2006.
16. The New drug abuse warning network report: emergency department visits involving patients with co-occurring disorders. Issue 15, 2006R.
17. Carise D, Dugosh KL, McLellen AT, et al. Prescription OxyContin abuse among patients entering addiction treatment. Am J Psychiatry 2007;164:1750–6.
18. Forman RF, Marlowe DB, McLellan AT. The Internet as a source of drugs of abuse. Curr Psychiatry Rep 2006;8:377–82.
19. National Center on Addiction and Substance Abuse at Columbia University. 'You've got drugs!', IV: prescription drug pushers on the Internet. A CASA white paper, 2007.
20. Greenberg PA. Report: online pharmacy sales top $1.9 billion. E-commerce times. Available at: www.ecommercetimes.com/story/2206.html. Accessed January 13, 2000.
21. Weiss AM. Buying prescription drugs on the Internet: promises and pitfalls. Cleve Clin J Med 2006;73(3):282–8.
22. Armstrong K, Schwartz JS, Asch DA. Direct sale of sildenafil (Viagra) to consumers over the Internet. N Engl J Med 1999;341:1389–92.
23. Young D. Experts warn drug industry, government about weaknesses in drug supply chain. Am J Health Syst Pharm 2003;60:2176–84.
24. Henney JE, Shuren JE, Nightingale SL, et al. Internet purchase of prescription drugs: buyer beware. Ann Intern Med 1999;131:861–2.
25. Hubbard WK. Testimony on Internet drug sales before the committee on government reform, house of representatives. Available at: www.hhs.gov/asl/testify/t040318.html. Accessed March 18, 2004.
26. Drug Enforcement Administration. Practitioner's manual: an informational outline of the controlled substances act of 1970. Washington, DC: US Dept of Justice, Office of Diversion Control; 2006.
27. US Dept of Justice, Office of the Inspector General, Evaluation and Inspections Division. Follow up review of the DEA's efforts to control the diversion of controlled pharmaceuticals, evaluation and inspections report I-2006-004. July 2006.
28. Joseph T. Rannazzisi, Deputy Assistant Administrator, Office of Diversion Control, DEA, US Dept of Justice, before the Subcommittee on Criminal Justice, Drug Policy and Human Resources. July 26, 2006.
29. Manchikanti L, Whitfield E, Pallone F. Evolution of the National All Schedules Prescription Electronic Reporting Act (NASPER): a public law for balancing treatment of pain and drug abuse and diversion. Pain Physician 2005;8:335–47.
30. Wang J, Christo P. The influence of prescription monitoring programs on chronic pain management. Pain Physician 2009;12:507–15.
31. Twillman R. Impact of prescription monitoring programs on prescription patterns and indicators of opioid abuse. J Pain 2006;7:S6.
32. Testimony of Nora D. Volkow, MD, Director, NIDA, NIH, US Dept of Health and Human Services, before the Subcommittee on Criminal Justice, Drug Policy, and Human Resources Committee. July 26, 2006.
33. Testimony of Sandra L. Kweder, MD, Deputy Director, Office of New Drugs Center for Drug Evaluation and Research, Food and Drug Administration, US Dept of

Health and Human Services, before the Subcommittee on Criminal Justice, Drug Policy and Human Resources. July 26, 2006.

34. Testimony of Stephen E. Johnson, Executive Director, Commercial Planning Pain Therapeutics, Inc. before the Subcommittee on Criminal Justice, Drug Policy and Human Resources. July 26, 2006.

35. Trescot AM, Helm S, Hansen H, et al. Opioids in the management of chronic non-cancer pain: an update of American Society of the Interventional Pain Physicians' (ASIPP) guidelines. Opioids Special Issue: Pain Physician 2009;11:S5–62.

36. International Association for the Study of Pain. Classification of chronic pain. Descriptions of chronic pain syndromes and definitions of pain terms. Pain Suppl 1986;3:S1–226.

37. Management of cancer pain. Management of cancer pain guideline panel. Clinical practice guideline no. 9. Rockville (MD): US Department of Health and Human Service, Public Health Service, Agency for Health Care Policy and Research; 1994. (AHCPR publication no. 94-0592).

38. Chou R, Fanciullo G, Fine P, et al. Clinical guidelines for the use of chronic opioid therapy in chronic noncancer pain. J Pain 2009;10:113–30.

39. Chou R. 2009 clinical guidelines from the American Pain Society and the American Academy of Pain Medicine on the use of chronic opioid therapy in chronic noncancer pain. What are the key messages for clinical practice? Pol Arch Med Wewn 2009;119(7–8):469–77.

40. Michna E, Ross EL, Hynes WL, et al. Predicting aberrant drug behavior in patients treated for chronic pain: importance of abuse history. J Pain Symptom Manage 2004;28(3):250–8.

41. Michna E, Jamison RN, Pharm LD, et al. Urine toxicology screening among chronic pain patients on opioid therapy: frequency and predictability of abnormal finding. Clin J Pain 2007;23:173–9.

42. Manubay JM, Comer SD, Sullivan MA. Treatment selection in substance abusers with pain. Adv Pain Manage 2008;2(2):59–67.

43. Gourlay DL, Heit HA, Almahrezi A. Universal precautions in pain medicine: a rational approach to the treatment of chronic pain. Pain Med 2005;6: 107–12.

44. Passik SD, Kirsh KL, Whitcomb L, et al. A new tool to assess and document pain outcomes in chronic pain patients receiving opioid therapy. Clin Ther 2004;26: 552–61.

45. Jaffe J. Opiates: clinical aspects. In: Lowinson J, Ruiz P, Mullman R, editors. Substance abuse: a comprehensive textbook. Baltimore (MD): Williams & Wilkins; 1992. p. 186–94.

46. Portenoy RK, Payne R. Acute and chronic pain. In: Lowinson J, Ruiz P, Millman R, et al, editors. Substance abuse: a comprehensive textbook. Baltimore (MD): Williams & Wilkins; 1997. p. 563–90.

47. Chou R, Clark E, Helfand M. Comparative efficacy and safety of long-acting oral opioids for chronic non-cancer pain; a systematic review. J Pain Symptom Manage 2003;26:1026–48.

48. Center for Substance Abuse Treatment. Methadone-associated mortality: report of a national assessment, 2003. Rockville (MD): Center for Substance Abuse Treatment, SAMHSA; 2004.

49. Reed JL, Ghodse AH. Oral glucose tolerance and hormonal response in heroin-dependent males. Br Med J 1973;2:582–5.

50. Willenbring ML, Morely JE, Krahn DD, et al. Psychoneuroendocrine effects of methadone maintenance. Psychoneuroendocrinology 1989;14(5):371–9.

51. Sullivan SN, Lee MG, Bloom SR, et al. Reduction by morphine of human postprandial insulin release is secondary to inhibition of gastrointestinal motility. Diabetes 1986;35(3):324–8.
52. Mehendale SR, Yuan CS. Opioid-induced gastrointestinal dysfunction. Dig Dis 2006;24:105–12.
53. Butler SF, Budman SH, Fernandez KC, et al. Development and validation of the current opioid misuse measure. Pain 2007;130:144–56.
54. Pereira J, Lawlor P, Vigano A, et al. Equianalgesic dose ratios for opioids: a critical review and proposals for long-term dosing. J Pain Symptom Manage 2001;22:672–8.
55. Fishbain DA, Cutler RB, Rosomoff HL, et al. Are opioid-dependent/tolerant patients impaired in driving-related skills? a structured evidence-based review. J Pain Symptom Manage 2003;25:559–77.
56. Patient-Centered Primary Care Collaborative. Patient centered medical home, patient centered primary care in the US. Patient-centered primary care collaborative 2007. Available at: www.pcpcc.net. Accessed April 1, 2010.

Alcohol Use Screening and Case Finding: Screening Tools, Clinical Clues, and Making the Diagnosis

John R. Freedy, MD, PhD[a],*, Katherine Ryan, BA[b]

KEYWORDS

- Screening • Case finding • Alcohol use disorders
- Screening and brief intervention

This article presents an evidence-based approach to screening (ie, universal assessment of all members of a group) and case finding (ie, selective assessment of only the group members at an increased risk) for alcohol use disorders in primary care. Problematic alcohol use by both adults and adolescents is considered. For clarity, this evidence-based presentation is divided into 6 sections: (1) epidemiology of alcohol use disorders, (2) associated health problems, (3) US Preventive Services Task Force (USPSTF) screening recommendations, (4) screening/case finding instruments, (5) screening/case finding strategies, and (6) summary. This article reviews state-of-the-art, evidence-based concepts and practices for screening and case finding for alcohol use disorders among adults and adolescents in primary care settings.

EPIDEMIOLOGY

It is important to clearly define the level of alcohol use of clinical interest. For example, more than 90% of American adults have ever used alcohol (approximately two-thirds currently use alcohol), and approximately 90% of high school students have used alcohol. However, most people who use alcohol do not suffer lasting adverse consequences.[1] Screening and case finding should assist the health care provider in finding patients who are either at risk for adverse consequences (hazardous or

[a] Department of Family Medicine, Medical University of South Carolina, 295 Calhoun Street, Charleston, SC 29401, USA
[b] Department of Psychiatry and Behavioral Sciences, Medical University of South Carolina, 67 President Street, Charleston, SC 29425, USA
* Corresponding author.
E-mail address: freedyjr@musc.edu

Prim Care Clin Office Pract 38 (2011) 91–103
doi:10.1016/j.pop.2010.11.007   **primarycare.theclinics.com**
0095-4543/11/$ – see front matter © 2011 Elsevier Inc. All rights reserved.

at-risk drinking) or already suffering adverse consequences because of their drinking behavior (alcohol abuse or dependence).[2] **Box 1** lists the currently accepted definitions of clinically relevant alcohol use. As implied in these definitions, an increase in the frequency, amount, or duration of alcohol consumption may be associated with a greater likelihood of adverse physical and mental health consequences.[1,2]

Most US adults have consumed alcohol at some point in their lives, and about one-third have engaged in hazardous or at-risk drinking at some time.[1,3] Of key importance, hazardous drinking is associated with several adverse physical and mental health outcomes (eg, accidents, injuries, legal problems, medical visits, illicit drug use, alcohol abuse or dependence, depression, anxiety, social conflicts, elevated blood pressure, and gastritis). Most importantly, screening and brief intervention (SBI) for hazardous drinking in primary care settings has been associated with sustained reductions in both drinking and adverse outcomes.[1,2,5–10] Prevalence of alcohol abuse and dependence among general US adults is as follows: 4.7% past year abuse, 17.8% lifetime abuse, 3.8% past year dependence, and 12.5% lifetime dependence.[11] Rates of alcohol use problems (ie, hazardous drinking, abuse, or dependence) are thought to be higher in primary care and other treatment-seeking samples than among general population samples.[3,5]

Substance use in adolescence is associated with an increased risk of alcohol dependence in adulthood. Lifetime prevalence rates of alcohol abuse generally increase across the teenage years, with a peak of 9.8% in the age range of 17 to 19 years. It is alarming to note that only about 10% of adolescents with alcohol abuse or dependence receive treatment.[12] Adolescents seen in primary care or other medical settings (for any reason) are more likely than general population teens to suffer alcohol abuse problems. Although only limited data are available, brief interventions based on motivational interviewing and similar cognitive behavioral strategies are promising in reducing the negative outcomes associated with adolescent drinking

---

Box 1
Alcohol use definitions

Alcohol use

    Any use of alcohol (standard drink is defined as 12 oz regular beer, 8 oz malt liquor, 5 oz table wine, 3.4 oz fortified wine, or 1.5 oz 80-proof liquor)[1]

Hazardous or at-risk drinking

    Alcohol consumption that confers the risk of physical and/or psychological harm (for men: ≥4 drinks at 1 time or >14 drinks weekly; for women: ≥3 drinks at 1 time or >7 drinks weekly)[1,3]

Alcohol abuse

    Maladaptive substance use leading to clinically significant impairment within a 12-month period (eg, role impairment because of substance use, recurrent substance use in hazardous situations, alcohol-related legal problems, or social problems caused or exacerbated by alcohol use)[4]

Alcohol dependence

    Maladaptive substance use leading to clinically significant impairment within a 12-month period, with 3 or more of the following occurring at any time in the 12-month period: tolerance, withdrawal, increased consumption, unsuccessful cutting down, great deal of time spent trying to obtain alcohol, important life activities given up for alcohol, or continued use despite knowledge of alcohol-related problems[4]

(eg, reduced alcohol use, increased treatment engagement, fewer emergency department (ED) visits, fewer accidents, and fewer legal consequences).[13]

ASSOCIATED HEALTH PROBLEMS

Problematic alcohol use is associated with a range of negative health issues among adults. Various forms of accidental injury and death are alcohol related (eg, 40% of traffic fatalities, one-third of ED trauma cases, increased boating accidents and accidental drowning, and increased interpersonal violence). Alcohol-related physical health problems include hypertension, myocardial infarction, heart failure, peptic ulcer disease, liver cirrhosis, malnutrition, various forms of cancer (mouth, esophagus, pharynx, larynx, liver, and breast cancer in women), upper respiratory tract infections, other minor infections because of impaired immune function, pneumonia, tuberculosis, pancreatitis, peripheral neuropathy, impaired sexual performance, fetal alcohol syndrome, falls with associated injuries, dementia, and delerium.[1,2,14] It seems that an increased level of daily alcohol consumption (for men, >4 drinks daily; for women, >2 drinks daily) is associated with increased mortality.[15] The following mental health problems have been associated with heavy alcohol use among adults: depression, bipolar disorder, other psychotic disorders, anxiety disorders (including posttraumatic stress disorder), and suicide.[1,16–22] The cost of care is substantially increased among problem drinkers when the patient suffers 1 or more comorbid mental health problems.[23]

Adolescents may also face several adverse consequences because of excess alcohol use. Nearly half of high school students report drinking alcohol within 30 days, and more than 40% of adolescents who report recent alcohol consumption admit binge drinking (≥5 drinks at a time). Among teenagers, this form of heavy alcohol consumption increases with each year of additional age. Frequency of adolescent binge drinking is positively associated with a range of negative health behaviors (eg, poor school performance, riding in a car with a driver who was drunk, sexual activity, smoking, illicit drug use, dating violence, and mental health problems). Youth drinking is also associated with the 3 leading causes of death from 12 to 20 years: unintentional injury, homicide, and suicide.[24] Among teenagers with substance abuse or dependence, up to three-fourths have a comorbid mental health problem (eg, depression, bipolar disorder, other psychotic disorders, anxiety disorder [including posttraumatic stress disorder], conduct disorder, oppositional defiant disorder, attention-deficit/hyperactivity disorder, and suicidal tendency). It is remarkable to note that about one-third of adolescents recall being asked about substance use, but two-thirds report a desire to discuss substance use with their primary care physician.[12]

The complex cause of adolescent alcohol use (particularly problematic use) merits special comment. Many personal, family, and community factors may influence adolescent alcohol use decisions. Examples of personal factors include developmental issues (delayed behavioral, emotional, or cognitive development), low self-esteem, or mental health issues (eg, depression and anxiety). Potential family factors might include a family history of substance abuse (both learned and genetic contributions), poor parenting skills, and childhood abuse or neglect.[12,13] Regarding biologic risk, it is thought that the reward pathways in the adolescent brain involving dopamine, serotonin, and norepinephrine may be particularly vulnerable to alcohol or other drugs, having an excessively reinforcing effect that may underlie the neurophysiology of addiction.[12] Community factors may include peer pressure or cultural factors (eg, identification with one's ethnic group has been associated with improved substance abuse treatment outcomes).[12,13]

Regardless of the precise cause, only about 10% of adolescents become problem drinkers as adults. In terms of risk stratification, it is worth noting that teenagers using alcohol before age 15 years are 5-fold more likely to develop adult alcohol abuse or dependence compared with teenagers who start alcohol use at age 21 years or later. Adolescents who demonstrate either substance abuse or dependence are also more likely to have similar problems as adults.[12] Extending this risk argument to college populations, 40% of college students report binge drinking ($\geq$5 drinks at a single time) within 2 weeks, and within the past 12 months, 33% qualify for alcohol abuse and 6% for alcohol dependence. On a more encouraging note, several well-done studies have shown that a variety of brief screening and intervention (BSI) efforts with binge drinking college students has resulted in desired outcomes (eg, reduced drinking and reduced harmful consequences). The following program elements have been shown to be useful: brief, personalized, motivational interviewing principles, real-time contact, no-contact approaches (written materials or computerized), and voluntary or mandatory participation. Follow-up periods for effective BSI programs among college students have ranged from several months to 4 years.[24]

USPSTF SCREENING RECOMMENDATIONS

In keeping with an evidence-based approach to screening and case finding for alcohol use disorders in primary care, this article reviews the USPSTF recommendations regarding screening for and treatment of alcohol use disorders among adults and adolescents in primary care. The USPSTF was established by the Agency for Health-care Research and Quality in 1984 as "an independent panel of experts in primary care and prevention that systematically review(s) the evidence of effectiveness and develops recommendations for clinical preventive services." At present, the USPSTF offers more than 100 evidence-based recommendations regarding screening and clinical interventions in primary care. As substantial new evidence accumulates, the USPSTF offers updated recommendations in each relevant area of clinical practice.[25] **Table 1** presents the current USPSTF recommendations regarding screening and behavioral counseling in primary care to reduce alcohol misuse.

The ability to translate the USPSTF recommendations into optimal clinical practice is well served by considering the nature of the USPSTF evidence reviews and recommendations. The USPSTF is a conservative body that thoroughly reviews the available evidence and, in particular, considers the strength (ie, quality and quantity) of the available evidence. This review includes a consideration of potential benefits, harms, and

Table 1
USPSTF alcohol misuse screening and behavioral counseling intervention recommendations
Adult recommendation
"The USPSTF recommends screening and behavioral counseling interventions to reduce alcohol misuse by adults, including pregnant women, in primary care settings." (Grade B recommendation)
Adolescent recommendation
"The USPSTF concludes that the evidence is insufficient to recommend for or against screening and behavioral counseling interventions to prevent or reduce alcohol misuse by adolescents in primary care settings." (Grade I statement)

Data from Screening and behavioral counseling interventions in primary care to reduce alcohol misuse, topic page. Rockville (MD): US Preventive Services Task Force. Agency for Healthcare Research and Quality; April 2004. Available at: http//www.ahrq.gov/clinic/uspstf/uspsdrin.htm. Accessed February 1, 2010.

the relative lack or paucity of evidence in a particular area of clinical practice. Accordingly, high recommendation levels (A: "... good evidence that the service improves important health outcomes and concludes that benefits substantially outweigh harms" or B: "... fair evidence that the service improves important health outcomes and concludes that benefits outweigh harms") are difficult to obtain. In fact, most Task Force recommendations are I statements.[25] An I statement does not mean that the service is not worth considering. In fact, competent clinicians (including Task Force members) may have an informed impression that an I statement service is worth doing at least in some circumstances (ie, leads to more potential benefit than risk of harm), but existing well-done research is insufficient (ie, too few studies to definitively conclude the likely benefit or definitively conclude the limited chance of harm) to reach the high threshold required to label the service with a more definitive recommendation (ie, level A or B recommendation).[25] At these instances, medical professionalism and the art of clinical practice require the provider to use professional judgment and to elicit values and priorities from the patient (or parents) in deciding the appropriateness of the level I service for a particular patient.

SCREENING/CASE FINDING INSTRUMENTS

The optimal selection and application of alcohol use screening or case finding instruments require an accurate understanding of the nature of primary care. In an ideal world, performing the core functions of primary care is daunting. These core functions include access (point of first contact), comprehensiveness (addressing most acute and chronic health care needs), continuity (continued care over time), and coordination (of multiple tests and services related to patient health). Increasingly, a variety of barriers (eg, numerous preventive services, complexity of medical conditions, loss of coverage or insurance restrictions that impair access, social expectations for immediate service, increasing documentation demands, and complexity of health care system making care coordination more difficult) make it difficult for primary care physicians to achieve these core functions.[26] Accordingly, only 13% of physicians routinely use alcohol screening questionnaires, and clinicians too often fail to make appropriate referrals based on positive screening results.[1]

Screening and case finding efforts should be implemented in such a way that the already overly pressurized primary care physician is not burdened. In addition to making limited time demands, screening and case finding efforts must be designed to enhance the quality of physician-patient relationships. This latter point is because most primary care physicians attain professional satisfaction with the relief of patient suffering through the skillful use of the physician-patient relationship.[27] It is also true that many primary care patients seek physicians who will listen empathically to their concerns without expecting the physician to solve all their problems.[28]

Time constraint is a major factor in the selection of alcohol screening or case finding tests for primary care. Instruments have evolved over time from standard-length screens (eg, 10-item Alcohol Use Disorders Identification Test [AUDIT]) to brief screens (4-item CAGE or 3-item AUDIT-C) to ultrabrief screens (single-item screen).[1,2,13] Each category of screening test has advantages and disadvantages. Furthermore, each type of screen can be used alone (single-stage screening) or with other screening instruments (2-stage or multistage screening).[29] Primary care alcohol use screening/case finding has evolved to the point that the major challenge is to develop an optimal integration of screening tests into primary care practice. This implementation science must meet both the practical (time limitations) and philosophic (enhancement of the quality of the physician-patient relationship) demands inherent in primary care practice.

An example of evidence-based ultrabrief screening for primary care is as follows: "On any single occasion during the past 3 months have you had more than 5 drinks containing alcohol?" It has been shown that a positive response to this single question may accurately identify primary care adult patients in the following alcohol consumption categories: hazardous/at-risk, alcohol abuse, and alcohol dependence.[30] A study of primary care adult patients showed 62% sensitivity (moderate false-negative results) and 93% specificity (minimal false-positive results) for hazardous or at-risk drinking for this single-item screen.[31] Fleming[30] has argued that stage 1 screening in primary care should involve the combination of an ultrabrief screening question (yes or no) and basic-level intervention involving a few brief physician statements (eg, "I am concerned about your drinking. The amount you are drinking exceeds recommended limits and could lead to alcohol-related problems. I'd like to recommend that you reduce your alcohol intake [or quit drinking]."). When applied to appropriate primary care populations (hazardous/at-risk drinkers primarily), the stage 1 SBI strategy has been shown to decrease drinking in both male and female adult patients of various ages.[30]

Brief screening instruments are typically used in what Fleming[30] refers to as stage 2 primary care screening. This level of screening can follow up "yes" responses to the previously cited ultrabrief screening question with the following 3 questions:

1. "On average, how many days per week do you drink alcohol?"
2. "On a typical day when you drink, how many drinks do you have?"
3. "What is the maximum number of drinks you had on any given day in the past month?"

Although stage 2 screening is more time consuming than stage 1 screening, it should be conducted annually for all adult patients. An intensified brief intervention is offered to patients meeting any of the following criteria: any binge drinking, men drinking more than 14 drinks weekly ($\geq$4 drinks daily), or women drinking more than 7 drinks weekly ($\geq$3 drinks daily). The conceptual goal of stage 2 screening is to increase sensitivity (reduce false-negative results) while maintaining suitably high specificity (minimal false-positive results). The intensified brief intervention includes 2 brief face-to-face physician interviews 1 month apart and a supportive, problem-focused telephone call 2 weeks after each face-to-face meeting (phone contacts can be made by the physician, nurse, or other designated clinical staff member). This intensified SBI led to positive results among primary care patients (primarily patients qualifying for hazardous or at-risk drinking and alcohol abuse) at a follow-up of up to 4 years (reduced alcohol use, fewer hospital days, and fewer ED visits).[30]

Standard-length screening instruments are used in what Fleming[30] describes as stage 3 screening. In essence, if stage 1 and 2 screenings suggest a potential alcohol problem (high sensitivity or minimal false-negative results and high specificity or minimal false-positive results regarding hazardous or at-risk drinking and alcohol abuse), then that patient is asked to complete a full-length screening instrument (eg, 10-item AUDIT). The research on AUDIT has suggested valid results with a variety of primary care populations (men, women, adolescents, adults, and less so with the elderly).[30] The AUDIT elicits quantitative responses to several areas that are important in better understanding the nature of a person's drinking behavior (quantity and frequency of drinking, frequency of binge drinking, dependence symptoms, and alcohol-related problems). Scores more than 8 represent a drinking behavior that exceeds healthy recommendations. Scores more than 16 are suggestive of either alcohol abuse or dependence.[14] Stage 3 brief intervention is further intensified and typically offered only to patients with either alcohol abuse or dependence problem, with the treatment goal of abstinence. The primary care physician or office-based mental health counselor provides cognitive-behaviorally oriented strategies to change the drinking behavior. Subspecialist referral is often included at this intervention level.[30]

Table 2 provides a summary of alcohol abuse screening tests that were cited as part of the evidence review used by the USPSTF in developing current recommendations regarding primary screening and intervention efforts.[34] A review of this table confirms that these screening tests were of the brief or full-length variety (no ultrabrief tests). A review of sensitivity (high sensitivity minimizes false-negative results) and specificity (high specificity minimizes false-positive results) confirms that no single test applied to primary care populations will eliminate case finding errors. The previously cited 3-stage screening/case finding process illustrates how combinations of screening/case finding tests (ultrabrief, brief, and full-length tests) can be used to promote optimal accuracy in clinical decision making (ie, to maximize sensitivity and specificity).[30]

Two additional alcohol screening tests merit comment for completeness. The AUDIT-C is a brief screen derived from the full-length AUDIT. It consists of 3 quantity questions:

1. "How often did you have a drink containing alcohol in the past year?"
2. "How many drinks did you have on a typical day when you were drinking in the past year?"
3. "How often did you have 6 or more drinks on 1 occasion in the past year?"

Using the same frequency scale from the full-length AUDIT, scores from 0 to 12 can be obtained on the AUDIT-C. Using various cut scores (2–5), adequate sensitivity (60%–94%) and specificity (56%–96%) can be obtained for adults engaged in various

Table 2
Alcohol misuse screening instruments from the USPSTF evidence review

Instrument	Population	Item No	Format	Sensitivity (%)	Specificity (%)
AUDIT[14]	Adults	10	Frequency	51–97	78–96
CAGE[32]	Adults	4	Yes/no	43–94	70–97
T-ACE[33]	Pregnant women	4	Yes/no and quantity	76	79
TWEAK[33]	Women	5	Yes/no and quantity	75–79	83–90
MAST-G[34]	Geriatrics	24	Yes/no	70	80
HSS[35]	Adults	10	Frequency	95–96	70–80

Abbreviations: AUDIT, Alcohol Use Disorders Identification Test; CAGE, C: have you every felt you should cut down on your drinking? (Cut down), A: have people annoyed you by criticizing your drinking? (Annoyed), G: have you ever felt bad or guilty about your drinking? (Guilty), E: have you ever had a drink first thing in the morning to steady your nerves or to get rid of a hang over? (Eye opener); HSS, Health Screening Survey; MAST-G (24 items), Michigan Alcoholism Screening Test-Geriatric Version; T-ACE, T: does it take more than three drinks to make you feel high? (Take), A: have you every been annoyed by people's criticism of your drinking? (Annoyed), C: are you trying to cut down on drinking? (Cut down), E: have you ever used alcohol as an eye opener in the morning? (Eye opener); TWEAK, T: how many drinks can you hold? (Tolerance), W: have close friends or relatives worried or complained about your drinking in the past year? (worried), E: do you sometimes take a drink in the morning when you first get up? (Eye opener), A: has a friend or family member every told you about things you said or did while you were drinking that you could not remember? (Amnesia), K: do you sometimes feel the need to cut down on your drinking? (K/cut down).

categories of harmful drinking (hazardous/at-risk drinking, alcohol abuse, and alcohol dependence).[35–37]

The CRAFFT questionnaire may be particularly useful with adolescents. The CRAFFT consists of the following (yes/no) items:

1. "Have you ever ridden in a *C*ar driven by someone (including yourself) who was 'high' or had been using alcohol or drugs?"
2. "Do you ever use alcohol or drugs to *R*elax, feel better about yourself, or fit in?"
3. "Do you ever use alcohol or drugs while you are by yourself, *A*lone?"
4. "Do you ever *F*orget things you did while using alcohol or drugs?"
5. "Do your family or *F*riends ever tell you that you should cut down on your drinking or drug use?
6. "Have you ever gotten into *T*rouble while you were using alcohol or drugs?"

A cut score of 2 or more among adolescents in primary care settings yielded 76% sensitivity and 94% specificity for any alcohol-related problem.[38] Research has suggested that other alcohol screening tests (eg, AUDIT and CAGE) should use lower cut scores when applied to samples comprising adolescents and college-aged adults.[1]

SCREENING/CASE FINDING STRATEGIES

Implementation science determines the best way to integrate a needed medical service into clinical practice. In this instance, the authors' interest is to improve the integration of alcohol use screening or case finding with adult or adolescent patients presenting in primary care settings. It is thought that this area of clinical practice will move forward in proportion to the degree to which the conceptual approach taken is ecologically valid for primary care practice. Screening efforts must save time and thus make it easier (not more difficult) for primary care physicians to address the core functions of primary care (access, comprehensiveness, continuity, and coordination).[26] Screening activities must also enhance the quality of the physician-patient relationship (eg, improved trust, quality of information exchanged, and quality of decisions made), or surely both providers and patients will reject screening/case finding and the associated intervention efforts.[27,28]

Implementation science has determined that mental health screening can save time for primary care providers. However, most primary care providers do not associate mental health screening (or other forms of screening) with time economy. That time saving is not only possible but also predictable is a point that needs to be taught to primary care physicians and their staff. Magruder and Yeager[29] have shown how predictable time economy may be associated with mental health screening in primary care. Most primary care physicians and their staff view time management in terms of an individual provider's schedule on a specific day (ie, "how many patients did we see today?"). However, the core functions of primary care call on physicians and their staff to manage populations at risk and not simply the individual patient. A more consequential idea is for the providers and their staff to consider the time saved (or lost) in providing an evidence-based clinical service (ie, the service should be more likely to provide benefit than harm) to a population of patients under their direct care (eg, all adults in a clinic panel). With this population-based perspective, it can be shown that mental health screening can be a time-saving practice.[29]

The following example illustrates this time economy point. Assuming a 5% prevalence for alcohol dependence, suppose that a single-stage screening approach (95% sensitivity and 60% specificity) is used. In the first step of screening, a high-sensitivity instrument is used to minimize the number of false-negative results (so as to not miss anyone with the condition of interest). In screening 1000 adult primary care patients from the authors' practice, 428 would screen positive, but only 50 would actually have alcohol dependence. This single-stage approach would lead to 380 false-positive cases, resulting in a diagnostic burden of 380/1000 (38%). If a second stage is added to this screening approach (2-stage screening; stage 2 sensitivity, 80%; specificity, 80%; higher specificity to remove false-positive cases), all 428 patients with a positive result in stage 1 screen are asked to complete the stage 2 screen. In stage 2, 114 patients screen positive, 314 screen negative, and the diagnostic burden decreases to 76 remaining false-positive results (76/428 or 17.8%). In considering time investment, the 2-stage approach saves time (per 1000 patients screened) for providers (20 minutes per positive screen for 77 hours for single-stage approach vs 38 hours for 2-stage approach), staff (2 minutes per positive screen for 33 hours for single-stage approach vs 14 hours for 2-stage approach), and patients (20 minutes per positive screen for 110 hours for single-stage approach vs 69 hours for 2-stage approach). It can also be demonstrated that with increased prevalence of alcohol dependence, time burden for providers, staff, and patients generally decreases further per 1000 patients tested (because of fewer false-positive results to evaluate).[29]

Implementation science can also be used to make the case that alcohol use screening or case finding can enhance the quality of the physician-patient relationship. By arguing in favor of a population-based approach (per 1000 patients screened), it is shown that providers, staff, and patients spend less time in screening activities. As a consequence, providers are free to spend their time performing clinical activities that are likely to have a meaningful effect on the patient's health and related quality of life.[27] The desire of primary care patients to see a physician who has the time to listen empathically to concerns is also well served through time efficiencies involved in staged screening efforts.[28]

An important concept in terms of enhancement of the quality of the physician-patient relationship is that alcohol screening activities must be designed into routine clinical practice (a function of the clinical care system, much like taking vital signs or tracking childhood immunizations). Based on the USPSTF recommendations, for adults (level B), all adults must be screened on an annual basis for possible alcohol problems.[25] For adolescents (level I), providers must use their clinical judgment and consider the individual circumstances (patients with higher risks being more likely to be assessed) in deciding when to screen for alcohol-related behaviors.[25] Primary care patients typically expect (and even welcome) inquiries about alcohol use or other health-related behaviors and report that providers assess such health behaviors less often than is considered to be desirable.[12] Systematizing such assessments may free providers to tend to more important aspects of the physician-patient relationship (eg, building trust, assessment of motivation or barriers, and management of other health-related behaviors or outcomes).

A discussion of systematizing the search for alcohol problems among primary care patients would not be complete without a consideration of the potential role for electronic medical records (EMRs). At present, less than 20% of practicing primary care providers use EMRs.[39] However, political, cultural, and economic trends are such that the use of EMRs is considered state-of-the-art and will only continue to grow.[40] Some have argued that barriers to effective EMR implementation and use can be overcome with time and specific strategies (eg, attending to computer literacy, dedicated time for EMR implementation and adoption, training activities, and support for information technology [IT] problem solvers within a practice).[41] On this point, a robust research literature concerning the role of computer-based assessment and medical practice exists. Many current EMRs have functions that allow for medical history taking to be done online before the patient sees the provider (patient completes questions with minimal assistance, or staff can enter responses for the patient, depending on how the system is designed).[42] With proper IT support, a provider (or provider group) could easily develop a health screening system (eg, based on the selected USPSTF screening recommendations, including alcohol-related behaviors) to be implemented through the EMR. The patient's chart could be flagged for the attention of the provider or staff only when the EMR function had removed the maximum number of patients with false-negative (high sensitivity) and false-positive (high specificity) results (staged screening could be programmed into the EMR, with step 1 involving a high-sensitivity test and step 2 involving a high-specificity test). The time of all involved (provider, staff, and patient) would be optimally used. Providers would be free to focus professional time on both the core functions of primary care (access, comprehensiveness, continuity, and coordination) and efforts to enhance the quality of the physician-patient relationship (building trust, assessment of motivation or barriers, and management of other health-related behaviors or outcomes). Patients would receive high-quality service based on the evidence-based guidelines for screening and intervention and would have an increased opportunity to be listened to empathically by a less-rushed primary care provider.[42]

SUMMARY

This article provides an evidence-based summary of screening (ie, universal assessment of all members of a group) and case finding (ie, selective assessment of only group members at increased risk) for alcohol use disorders among adults and adolescents in primary care. Key concepts are reviewed to illustrate state-of-the-art, evidence-based concepts and practices. The following areas were summarized:

- Although most adults (90%) and adolescents (>90% by high school graduation) have consumed alcohol, many adults and adolescents never develop problems related to alcohol use.
- The focus of alcohol screening and case finding efforts should be on finding adult and adolescent primary care patients with clinically relevant forms of alcohol use (hazardous or at-risk drinking, alcohol abuse, or alcohol dependence) that have been associated with adverse patient outcomes.
- Among adults, the following lifetime rates of clinically relevant alcohol use exist: 33% at-risk or hazardous drinking, 17.8% alcohol abuse, and 12.5% alcohol dependence.
- Among adolescents, binge drinking is reported among 40% who drank in the past 30 days, and alcohol abuse increases with age, with a peak of 9.8% in the age range of 17 to 19 years.
- Rates of clinically relevant drinking are generally considered to be higher among patients seeking primary care or other medical services than among adults or adolescents in the general population.
- Adults may experience alcohol-related health issues that range from mild (eg, hypertension or gastritis) to severe (eg, accidental injuries or death, various forms of cancer, or premature mortality).
- Adolescents may experience alcohol-related health issues that range from mild (eg, poor school performance or riding in a car with someone who has been drinking) to severe (eg, dating violence, mental health problems, or death).
- Research on BSI for adults and adolescents attending primary care medical appointments suggests that this approach produces several positive outcomes

likely to mitigate both mild and severe health issues that might otherwise be associated with clinically relevant forms of alcohol use.

- The USPSTF suggests that there is fair evidence (B recommendation) to support screening and behavioral counseling interventions for adults in primary care.
- The USPSTF suggests that there is insufficient evidence (I recommendation) to support screening and behavioral counseling interventions for adolescents in primary care. Nevertheless, based on professional judgment and the clinical art of medicine, primary care physicians can choose to screen for clinically relevant forms of alcohol use among adolescents thought to be at increased risk for alcohol-related problems (case finding approach).
- Screening/case finding instruments have evolved over time to meet both the practical (time limits) and philosophic (promoting the primary care core functions of access, comprehensiveness, continuity, and coordination as a means to enhance the quality of the physician-patient relationship) demands of primary care practice. Three lengths of screening tests exist (ultrabrief or 1 item, brief or 6 items or less, and standard length or 10–20 items). In practice, 2-stage or multistage screening/case findings can be used to produce maximally accurate results. Brief intervention efforts can be systematically intensified according to the level of suspected alcohol use inferred from testing results (hazardous or at-risk drinking, alcohol abuse, or alcohol dependence).
- Screening strategies involve what the authors have termed implementation science. Screening/case finding efforts with regard to alcohol use among adults and adolescents in primary care can be improved to the extent that the conceptual approach is ecologically valid for primary care practice. The authors particularly advocate the following key concepts: primary care physicians and staff must begin to look at screening/case finding efforts as an effort to better manage populations at risk and not simply an individual patient; using a 2-stage approach (sensitivity, >90% for stage 1; sensitivity/specificity, 80%/80% for stage 2), time saving per 1000 patients assessed can be demonstrated for providers, staff, and patients. Furthermore, increasing the prevalence among the patient population results in increased time saving for providers, staff, and patients per 1000 patients in a predictable fashion.
- Implementation science should capitalize on EMR technology in designing staged screening protocols with the goal of minimizing false-negative and false-positive results among cases flagged for additional provider or staff attention. Implementing this use of EMR technology should carefully address potential barriers to success (eg, addressing computer literacy, dedicated time for EMR implementation and adoption, training activities, and support for IT problem solvers within a practice).

REFERENCES

1. Gold MS, Aronson MD. Screening for and diagnosis of alcohol problems. 2009. Reprint from UptoDate. Topic last updated. Available at: www.utdol.com/online/content/topic.do?topicKey=subabuse/8392&;view=print. Accessed February 15, 2010.
2. DynaMed Summary. Alcohol use disorder. Available at: www.dynaweb.ebscohost.com/Detail.aspz?id=115540&;sid=fc860746–43b5-4b98-aa3a-1cef4f293280%4. Accessed March 1, 2010.

3. Feldman MD, Christensen JF, editors. Behavioral medicine: a guide for clinical practice. 3rd edition. New York: The McGraw-Hill Companies, Inc; 2008.

4. American Psychiatric Association. Diagnostic and statistical manual of mental disorders. text revision. 4th edition. Washington, DC: American Psychiatric Association; 2000.

5. McQuade WH, Levy SM, Yanek LR, et al. Detecting symptoms of alcohol abuse in primary care settings. Arch Fam Med 2000;9:814–21.

6. Madras BK, Compton WM, Avula D, et al. Screening, brief interventions, referral to treatment (SBIRT) for illicit drug and alcohol use at multiple healthcare sites: comparison at intake and 6 months later. Drug Alcohol Depend 2009;99:280–95.

7. Kaner E, Bland M, Cassidy P, et al. Screening and brief interventions for hazardous and harmful alcohol use in primary care: a cluster randomized controlled trial protocol. BMC Public Health 2009;9:287.

8. Nilsen P. Brief alcohol intervention—where to from here? Challenges remain for research and practice. Addiction 2010;105(6):954–9.

9. Solberg LI, Maciosek MV, Edwards NM. Primary care intervention to reduce alcohol misuse: ranking its health impact and cost effectiveness. Am J Prev Med 2008;34(2):143–52.

10. Babor TF, Higgins-Biddle J, Dauser D, et al. Alcohol screening and brief intervention in primary care settings: implementation models and predictors. J Stud Alcohol 2005;66:361–8.

11. Hasin DS, Stinson FS, Ogburn E, et al. Prevalence, correlates, disability, and comorbidity of DSM-IV alcohol abuse and dependence in the United States: results from the National Epidemiologic Survey on Alcohol and Related Conditions. Arch Gen Psychiatry 2007;64(7):830–42.

12. Griswold KS, Aronoff H, Kernan JB, et al. Adolescent substance use and abuse: recognition and management. Am Fam Physician 2008;77(3):331–6.

13. Ries RK, Miller SC, Fiellin DA, et al, editors. Principles of addiction medicine. 4th edition. Philadelphia: Wolters Kluwer/Lippincott Williams & Wilkins; 2009.

14. Babor TB, Higgins-Biddle JC, Saunders JB, et al. The alcohol use disorders identification test: guidelines for use in primary care. 2nd edition. Geneva (Switzerland): World Health Organization Department of Mental Health and Substance Dependence; 2001.

15. Castelnuovo AD, Costanzo S, Bagnardi V, et al. Alcohol dosing and total mortality in men and women. Arch Intern Med 2006;166:2437–45.

16. Ries RK. Co-occurring alcohol use and mental disorders. J Clin Psychopharmacol 2006;26(s1):30–6.

17. Frye MA, Salloum IM. Bipolar disorder and comorbid alcoholism: prevalence rate and treatment considerations. Bipolar Disord 2006;8:677–85.

18. Kessler RC. The epidemiology of dual diagnosis. Biol Psychiatry 2004;56:730–7.

19. Kushner MG, Abrams K, Borchard C. The relationship between anxiety disorders and alcohol use disorders: a review of major perspectives and findings. Clin Psychol Rev 2000;20(2):149–71.

20. Brown PJ, Recupero PR, Stout R. PTSD substance abuse comorbidity and treatment utilization. Brief report. Addict Behav 1995;20(2):251–4.

21. Mancebo MC, Grant JE, Pinto A, et al. Substance use disorders in an obsessive compulsive disorder clinical sample. J Anxiety Disord 2009;23:429–35.

22. Blume AW, Resor MR, Villanueva MR, et al. Alcohol use and comorbid anxiety, traumatic stress, and hopelessness among Hispanics. Addict Behav 2009;34:709–13.

23. Dickey B, Azeni H. Persons with dual diagnoses of substance abuse and major mental illness: their excess costs of psychiatric care. Am J Public Health 1996;86:973–7.

24. Miller JW, Naimi TS, Brewer RD, et al. Binge drinking and associated health risk behaviors among high school students. Pediatrics 2007;119:76–85.
25. Screening and behavioral counseling interventions in primary care to reduce alcohol misuse, topic page. Rockville (MD): US Preventive Services Task Force. Agency for Healthcare Research and Quality; 2004. Available at: http://www.ahrq.gov/clinic/uspstf/uspsdrin.htm. Accessed February 22, 2010.
26. Grumbach K, Bodenheimer T. A primary care home for Americans: putting the house in order. JAMA 2002;288(7):889–93.
27. Fairhurst K, May C. What general practitioners find satisfying in their work: implications for health care system reform. Ann Fam Med 2006;4(6):500–5.
28. Freedy JR, Magruder KM, Zoller JS, et al. Traumatic events and mental health in civilian primary care: implications for training and practice. Fam Med 2010;42(3): 185–92.
29. Magruder KM, Yeager DE. Screening for depression in primary care: can it become more efficient? In: Mitchel AJ, Coyne JC, editors. Screening for depression in clinical practice: an evidence-based guideline. New York: Oxford University Press; 2010. p. 161–90.
30. Fleming MF. Screening and brief intervention in primary care setting. Alcohol Res Health 2005;28(3):57–62.
31. Fiellin DA, Reid MC, O'Connor PG. Screening for alcohol problems in primary care: a systemic review. Arch Intern Med 2000;160(13):1977–89.
32. Russell M. New assessment tools for risk drinking during pregnancy: T-ACE, TWEAK, and others. Alcohol Health Res World 1994;18(1):55–61.
33. Fleming MF, Barry KL. A three-sample test of a masked alcohol screening questionnaire. Alcohol Alcohol 1991;26(1):81–91.
34. US Preventive Services Task Force. Evidence syntheses, formerly systematic evidence reviews. Screening instruments. Available at: www.ncbi.nlm.gov/bookshelf/br.fcgi?book=hsevidsyn&;part=A45594. Accessed March 2010.
35. Bush K, Kivlahan DR, McDonell MB, et al. The AUDIT alcohol consumption questions (AUDIT-C): an effective brief screening test for problem drinking. Ambulatory Care Quality Improvement Project (ACQUIP). Alcohol use disorders identification test. Arch Intern Med 1998;158(16):1789–95.
36. Gordon AJ, Maisto SA, McNeil N, et al. Three questions can detect hazardous drinkers. J Fam Pract 2001;50(4):313–20.
37. Bradley KA, Bush KR, Epler AJ, et al. Two brief alcohol-screening tests from the Alcohol Use Disorders Identification Test (AUDIT): validation in a female veterans affairs patient population. Arch Intern Med 2003;163(7):821–9.
38. Knight JR, Sherritt L, Shrier LA, et al. Validity of the CRAFFT substance abuse screening test among adolescent clinic patients. Arch Pediatr Adolesc Med 2002;156:607–14.
39. Loomis GA, Ries JS, Saywell RM Jr, et al. If electronic medical records are so great, why aren't family physicians using them? J Fam Pract 2002;51(7):636–41.
40. Dawes M, Chan D. Knowing we practise good medicine: implementing the electronic medical record in family practice [commentary]. Can Fam Physician 2010; 56(1):15–6.
41. Terry AL, Giles G, Brown JB, et al. Adoption of electronic medical records in family practice: the providers' perspective. Fam Med 2009;41(7):508–12.
42. Bachman JW. The patient-computer interview: a neglected tool that can aid the clinician. Mayo Clin Proc 2003;78:67–78.

Brief Interventions for Alcohol Misuse

Rick Botelho, MD[a],*, Brett Engle, PhD[b],
Jorge Camilo Mora, MD, MPH[c], Cheryl Holder, MD[d]

KEYWORDS

- Alcohol • AUDIT • Dependency • At-risk alcohol use

EVIDENCE-BASED BRIEF INTERVENTIONS

Alcohol misuse harms individuals and society with massive biopsychosocial and economic consequences: decreased worker productivity, increased unintentional injuries, aggression and violence against others, and child and spouse abuse (http://pubs.niaaa.nih.gov/publications/arh27-1/52-62.htm). The US Preventive Services Task Force recommends brief interventions for reducing alcohol misuse by adults, including pregnant women.[1] Brief counseling improves health outcomes, with the benefits outweighing the harms. However, the number, quality, and consistency in these studies limit the strength of the evidence. Brief interventions are effective in primary care settings, emergency departments, and college student health centers.[2–5] A review of a 22-study meta-analysis (7619 participants) showed that a brief intervention delivered to patients in primary care settings resulted in lower alcohol consumption (mean difference, −38 g/week, 95% confidence interval, −54 to −23) compared with controls.[1] Another review of a 19-study meta-analysis (5639 participants) showed that a brief intervention reduced alcohol consumption by 10% to 30%.[2] In a college student health center study, students who were screened positive for high-risk drinking reduced their alcohol consumption, with fewer peak number of drinks per sitting (control [C], 8.03; intervention [I], 6) and decrease in blood alcohol levels at 3 and 6 months (C, 0.071; I, 0.057 and C, 0.073; I, 0.057, respectively).

Although brief interventions are effective for certain populations, they have many limitations. They may or may not work with adolescents and do not conclusively reduce alcohol consumption in women and in heavy alcohol users in hospitals and primary care settings.[1,4,6] In drinkers with Alcohol Use Disorders Identification Test

[a] University of Rochester, Rochester Center to Improve Communication in Health Care, Building Relationships, Eliminating Disparities, 1381 South Clinton, Rochester, NY 14620, USA
[b] Barry University, 11300 NE Second Avenue, Miami Shores, FL 33161, USA
[c] Department of Humanities, Health & Society, Herbert Wertheim College of Medicine, Florida International University, 11200 SW 8th Street, HLSII 491, Miami, FL 33199, USA
[d] Department of Humanities, Health and Society, Herbert Wertheim College of Medicine, Florida International University Miami, FL 33199, USA
* Corresponding author.
E-mail address: RBotelho@me.com

Prim Care Clin Office Pract 38 (2011) 105–123
doi:10.1016/j.pop.2010.11.008
0095-4543/11/$ – see front matter © 2011 Published by Elsevier Inc.

primarycare.theclinics.com

(AUDIT) scores less than 8 (borderline at-risk drinkers and below), brief interventions did not reduce the average number of drinks per week or the number of binge episodes (>4 standard drinks on one occasion for men and >3 standard drinks for women) as compared with those who did not receive an intervention.[6,7]

PREVENTION PARADOX

The expenditures for the treatment of alcohol dependency far exceed the investments to prevent alcohol problems, even though the negative health and economic impacts of at-risk and harmful drinking exceed the negative consequences of alcohol dependency.[8] Secondary prevention has a far greater potential of improving the overall health of the population than tertiary prevention.[9] The implementation of low-risk drinking limits (secondary prevention) would result in an estimated 14.2% and 47.1% reduction in the prevalence of alcohol abuse and dependency, respectively.[10]

To address this prevention paradox, health care organizations should develop systems of care and train practitioners to systematically introduce Screening Brief Interventions and Referral to Treatments (SBIRT) programs into mainstream clinical practice.[11] Practitioners can use the concept of the alcohol risk and harm reduction to implement SBIRT programs.

ALCOHOL RISK AND HARM REDUCTION

Practitioners can use this concept to guide the negotiation process with patients in making tentative and definitive diagnoses about at-risk drinking and the severity of problem drinking (alcohol abuse and dependence). They can advise and encourage patients to cut down on their drinking or abstain from alcohol as a short-term experiential learning process or as a long-term goal. The strategy underlying this concept is to lower the severity of the problems and potential negative consequences arising from heavy drinking (drinking more than low-risk drinking limits). The goal of using this concept is to reduce the overall percentage of patients who drink more than low-risk limits, whatever their severity of risk and harms. When it is not possible to achieve the ideal goal for change, practitioners can help patients make incremental reductions in their risks and harms associated with heavy drinking or drug use.

ALCOHOL RISK-AND-HARM CONTINUUM REDUCTION

The alcohol risk-and-harm continuum describes the spectrum of at-risk and problem drinking: abstinence, low-risk use, hazardous use, harmful use, or abuse of alcohol and alcohol dependence. The percentage of the population that suffers from alcohol abuse and dependence is approximately 15% to 20% and 5%, respectively.

Low-Risk Use

The US National Institute of Alcohol Abuse and Alcoholism (NIAAA) describes its recommendations for low-risk drinking limits for men and women in a physician's guide. Men are at risk for alcohol-related problems if they drink more than 14 standard drinks in a week or more than 4 standard drinks on 1 occasion. Nonpregnant women are considered to be at risk if they drink more than 7 drinks per week or more than 3 drinks on any 1 occasion. A standard drink is equivalent to 12 ounces of beer (5% alcohol), 5 ounces of wine (10%–12% alcohol), 3 ounces of fortified alcohol (18%–20% alcohol), and 1.5 ouncesof hard liquor (80 proof; 40% alcohol) (**Table 1**).

Table 1		
Weekly maximum alcohol consumption		
	United States	
Alcohol	**Men**	**Women**
Standard number of drinks	14	7
Grams per drink	12	12
Total grams per week	168	84

At-Risk Use

At-risk use of alcohol is defined as drinking more than low-risk limits without evidence of alcohol abuse or dependency. These patients are at an increased risk for developing alcohol abuse and dependency, particularly if they increase their consumption over time.

Abuse

Alcohol abuse is defined as drinking that causes any negative medical, psychological, and/or social consequences. **Box 1** and **Table 2** summarize the *Diagnostic and Statistical Manual of Mental Disorders* (Fourth Edition) (DSM-IV) classification for alcohol abuse, use, and dependency.

SCREENING

The World Health Organization Early Intervention Project developed the 10-item AUDIT questionnaire (**Fig. 1**) to detect at-risk and problem drinking in hospitals and primary care settings.[12] Patients can complete the AUDIT instrument before physician encounters by checking the answer to each question.

The CAGE questionnaire (**Table 3**) is a brief instrument that is used when practitioners suspect only alcohol dependence.[13] This questionnaire does not assess for at-risk drinking, and a negative response misses most patients with alcohol abuse.[14]

Take a Family History

Patients with a family history of substance abuse are at an increased risk of developing alcohol and drug problems. Family, twin, half-sibling, and adoption studies of

Box 1
DSM-IV alcohol abuse
A maladaptive pattern of alcohol use leading to clinically significant impairment or distress, as manifested by one (or more) of the following occurring within a 12-month period 1. Recurrent drinking resulting in a failure to fulfill major role obligations at work, school, or home 2. Recurrent drinking in situations in which it is physically hazardous 3. Recurrent alcohol-related legal problems 4. Continued alcohol use despite having persistent or recurrent social or interpersonal problems caused or exacerbated by the effects of alcohol The symptoms have never met the criteria for alcohol dependence

Table 2
DSM-IV definitions of abuse and dependence

Symptoms	A. A maladaptive pattern of alcohol use, leading to clinically significant impairment or distress, as manifested by 3 or more of the following occurring at any time in the same year:
Tolerance	1. Need for markedly increased amounts of alcohol to achieve intoxication or desired effect or markedly diminished effect with continued use of the same amount of alcohol
Withdrawal	2. Ahe characteristic withdrawal syndrome for alcohol or alcohol (or a closely related substance) is taken to relieve or avoid withdrawal symptoms
Impaired Control	3. Persistent desire or 1 or more unsuccessful efforts to cut down or control drinking 4. Drinking in larger amounts or over a longer period than the person intended
Neglect of Activities	5. Important social, occupational, or recreational activities given up or reduced because of drinking
Time Spent Drinking	6. A great deal of time spent in activities necessary to obtain alcohol, to drink, or to recover from its effects
Drinking Despite Problems	7. Continued drinking despite knowledge of having a persistent or recurrent physical or physiologic problem that is likely to be caused or exacerbated by alcohol use
Compulsive Use	None
Duration Criterion	B. No duration criterion separately specified. However, 3 or more dependence criteria must be met within the same year and must occur repeatedly, as specified by duration qualifiers associated with criteria (eg, "often," "persistent," "continued")
Criterion for Subtyping Dependence	With physiologic dependence: evidence of tolerance or withdrawal, ie, any of items A(1) or A(2) above are present Without physiologic dependence: no evidence of tolerance or withdrawal, ie, none of items A(1) or A(2) above are present

alcoholic subjects suggest that the risk of inheritance of alcoholism is 50% to 60%.[15] The questions can identify other family members who have drug or alcohol problems. For those patients whose family members have current alcohol or drug problems, practitioners can provide resource material to help them with referring their relatives to professional services (**Box 2**).

TAKING AN ALCOHOL HISTORY

The practitioner can use a prevention-focused or problem-focused approach to take an alcohol history. With a preventive approach, practitioners can ask direct questions about alcohol use in a nonjudgmental manner.

- What kinds of alcohol do you drink? Beer, wine, hard liquor?
- How many drinks do you have in a week?
- What size drinks do you usually have?
- How many bottles of beer, wine, or hard liquor do you buy in a week?

However, some patients view such neutral questions as an intrusion and become defensive and vague about their alcohol intake. Leading questions provide a positive

1. How often do you have a drink containing alcohol?				
Never	Monthly or less	Two to four times a month	Two to three times a week	Four or more times a week
2. How many drinks containing alcohol do you have on a typical day when you are drinking?				
1 or 2	3 or 4	5 or 6	7 to 9 10 or more	
3. How often do you have six or more drinks on one occasion?				
Never	Less than monthly	Monthly	Weekly	Daily or almost daily
4. How often during the last year have you found that you were not able to stop drinking once you had started?				
Never	Less than monthly	Monthly	Weekly	Daily or almost daily
5. How often during the last year have you failed to do what was normally expected from you because of drinking?				
Never	Less than monthly	Monthly	Weekly	Daily or almost daily
6. How often during the last year have you needed a first drink in the morning to get yourself going after a heavy drinking session?				
Never	Less than monthly	Monthly	Weekly	Daily or almost daily
7. How often during the last year have you had a feeling of guilt or remorse after drinking?				
Never	Less than monthly	Monthly	Weekly	Daily or almost daily
8. How often during the last year have you been unable to remember what happened the night before because you had been drinking?				
Never	Less than monthly	Monthly	Weekly	Daily or almost daily
9. Have you or someone else been injured as a result of your drinking?				
No	Yes, but not in the last year		Yes, during the last year	
10.Has a relative, friend, doctor or other health worker been concerned about your drinking or suggested you cut down?				
No	Yes, but not in the last year		Yes, during the last year	

Fig. 1. AUDIT questionnaire. Questions 1 to 8 are scored 0 to 4 points, and questions 9 to 10 are scored 0, 2, or 4 points, giving a possible range of 0 to 40 points.

Table 3 CAGE questionnaire	
C	"Have you ever felt you should Cut down on your drinking?"
A	"Has anyone Annoyed you by criticizing your drinking?"
G	"Have you ever felt bad or Guilty about your drinking?"
E	"Have you ever had a drink (an Eye-opener) first thing in the morning to steady your nerves or to get rid of a hangover?"

Decision rule: two or more positive responses indicate alcohol abuse or dependence.
  One positive response warrants further assessment.

frame by assuming that people enjoy drinking alcohol. Leading questions can often obtain a more accurate alcohol history.

- So what kinds of alcohol do you like to drink?
- What are your favorite drinks?
- What do you like to drink when you go out to a party?

With a problem-focused approach, practitioners can use prefacing statements and exploratory questions to explore how patients view the association between their presenting problems and alcohol use. Prefacing statements link the use of alcohol to patients' presenting complaints in ways that can also provide a rationale for conducting an assessment.

- Some people find that drinking alcohol helps them get to sleep. What is this like for you?
- Some people do not realize that drinking alcohol can make their stomach pain worse. Have you noticed any patterns between your use of alcohol and your stomach problem?

Exploratory questions help the practitioner engage patients in assessing how their health problems relate to their alcohol use.

- Has your stomach problem affected how much you drink?
- Has drinking alcohol made your depression feel better or worse?
- How does drinking alcohol affect your sleep?
- How is your sleeping problem affected by your use of alcohol?
- What concerns your family (spouse or children) about how your drinking affects your health?

EDUCATE PATIENTS ABOUT THE AUDIT RESULTS

The practitioner can use the elicit-provide-elicit framework to educate patients about the result of their AUDIT survey. A brief video demonstration of these skills is available at (https://webmeeting.nih.gov/tutorial/) (**Table 4**).

EDUCATE PATIENTS ABOUT LOW-RISK DRINKING LIMITS

The practitioner can use the elicit-provide-elicit framework to educate patients about low-risk drinking limits. A brief video demonstration of these skills is available at: https://webmeeting.nih.gov/tutorial/.

Table 4 Brief interventions	
Audit Score	
Score = 0–7	Advise patients to continue with low-risk drinking or abstinence
Score = 8–15	Educate and advice patients to reduce to below low-risk drinking limits
Score = 15–20	Counsel patients about the risks of alcohol abuse and dependence Advise patients to reduce to below low-risk drinking limits or abstain
Score = 20–40	As above and assess for degree of alcohol dependence. Negotiate a referral for a specialist evaluation if patients are willing

NEGOTIATING A TENTATIVE DIAGNOSIS

Given the time pressures and limitations in most practitioner-patient encounters, most patients with alcohol problems remain undetected by their practitioners, except in the obvious cases. Therefore, practitioners encounter challenges in making definitive diagnoses of alcohol abuse or alcohol dependence with a high degree of certainty.

The AUDIT questionnaire and alcohol use history can identify patients who drink more than the low-risk drinking limits. Practitioners can use the elicit-inform-elicit framework (as previously described) to develop a shared understanding about the diagnostic likelihood for at-risk drinking. They can educate patients about using a likelihood scale (possibly, probably, definitely) to reduce diagnostic uncertainty (**Table 5**). For example, the practitioner may suspect a range of possibilities about the likelihood and severity of patients' at-risk and problem drinking, but patients may believe that their alcohol use is normal.

Even when practitioners are certain of a diagnosis, it is often challenging to inform patients in ways that they will accept it. Instead of giving the patient a diagnostic label, practitioners can negotiate a shared understanding about the likelihood and the severity of the problem. In this way, they can use clinical uncertainty to negotiate a shared understanding about the likelihood of a diagnosis (**Box 3**).

Using the likelihood scale, the practitioner can educate patients about at-risk and problem drinking in a nonthreatening way. For example, "The amount you are drinking is definitely above low-risk limits. What I'm concerned about is that your alcohol is probably causing your high blood pressure." It is often easier to reach a consensus with patients about at-risk drinking than it is to gain agreement about alcohol dependence. Many patients are surprised that they drink more than most of the population.

Table 5 Address differences in perspective about alcohol use			
		Problem Drinker	
Likelihood of a Problem	**At-Risk Drinker (Hazardous Use)**	**Abuse**	**Dependency**
Definitely	Pr	—	—
Probably	—	Pr	—
Possibly	—	—	Pr
Unlikely	Pt	Pt	Pt

Abbreviations: Pr, practitioner's opinion; Pt, practitioner's opinion of patient's perspective.

Reproduced from Botelho RJ. Motivational practice: promoting healthy habits and self-care of chronic diseases. MHH Publications; 2004; with permission.

> **Box 3**
> **Using the likelihood scale to educate patients about their alcohol use**
>
> For hazardous drinking: "I'm concerned that you are (possibly, probably, definitely) drinking above what are considered to be low-risk limits. What do you think?" (Let the patient respond.)
>
> For harmful drinking: "I'm concerned that your health problems are (possibly, probably, definitely) caused (or are made worse) by your alcohol use. What do you think?" (Let the patient respond.)
>
> For alcohol dependence: "I'm concerned that you are (possibly, probably, definitely) dependent upon alcohol (or have built up a tolerance to the effects of alcohol) because.... What do you think?" (Let the patient respond.)
>
> *Reproduced from* Botelho RJ. Motivational practice: promoting healthy habits and self-care of chronic diseases. MHH Publications; 2004. Available at: www.MotivateHealthyHabits.com; with permission.

They may doubt, resist, and resent even a tentative diagnosis of alcohol abuse. Rather than argue about the diagnosis, practitioners can educate patients to gain some common ground about the likelihood of at-risk drinking and alcohol abuse (**Table 6**).

Thus, the practitioner and the patient reach common ground about probable hazardous use and possible abuse of alcohol. However, they disagree on the possibility of alcohol dependence. Practitioners can focus on this common ground to select interventions that patients are willing to accept. If patients resist reaching common ground about the possibility of alcohol abuse, practitioners can invite patients to abstain from alcohol for a while to see if their medical or psychological problems resolve or become less severe. Before recommending a trial of abstinence, practitioners can assess for past withdrawal symptoms, particular if they suspect that the patient has a risk of alcohol dependence.

BRIEF EDUCATION AND ADVICE INTERVENTIONS

These materials are based on NIAAA publications that provide a video introduction to brief interventions (Video: Helping Patients Who Drink Too Much, https://webmeeting.nih.gov/tutorial/) (Appendix 1).

Table 6
Enhance mutual understanding about alcohol use

	At-Risk Drinker	Problem Drinker	
Likelihood of a Problem	Hazardous Use	Abuse	Dependency
Definitely	—	—	—
Probably	C	—	—
Possibly	—	C	Pr
Unlikely	—	—	Pt

Abbreviations: C, common agreement between practitioner and patient; Pr, practitioner's opinion; Pt, patient's opinion.

Reproduced from Botelho RJ. Motivational practice: promoting healthy habits and self-care of chronic diseases. MHH Publications; 2004; with permission.

Box 4
Enhancing mutual understanding about alcohol use provides stage-specific rationale

Precontemplation: You think that alcohol is helping your sleep (or depression), but in fact, it makes it worse. Can we use a decision balance so I could understand better the other reasons why you like to drink?

Contemplation: You are uncertain about whether alcohol is causing (or making worse) your stomach problem, hypertension, or any other medical problem. Some people find it helpful to do what is called a decision balance to help decide what to do. One option could be to cut down to low-risk drinking limits. Another could be to quit drinking for a trial period to see if your health problem gets better.

Reproduced from Botelho RJ. Motivational practice: promoting healthy habits and self-care of chronic diseases. MHH Publications; 2004. Available at: www.MotivateHealthyHabits.com; with permission.

USE THE STAGES OF CHANGE WITH A DECISION BALANCE

To address whether to abstain from alcohol or reduce to low-risk drinking limits, practitioners can provide a stage-specific rationale for using a decision balance, particularly with patients who are not thinking about change and those who are thinking about a change but ambivalent about it (**Boxes 4** and **5**).

Practitioners can ask the questions in the sequence suggested in **Table 7**.

After completing the decision balance, practitioners give a copy of the decision balance to the patient and keep another in the patient's records. Alternatively, patients can fill out the decision balance in the waiting room or as a homework assignment for the next visit, perhaps with the input of a family member.

The decision balance helps practitioners to understand the patients' reasons to drink and their reason to cut down or abstain from the patients' perspective. Such an understanding can help practitioners be more effective in gaining patients' cooperation in exploring how alcohol affects their health, family, work, and other aspects of life.

Once the decision balance is completed, the patients may be asked to score how important their reasons are to stay the same (resistance score) and to change (motivation score), using the questions below. Then patients can monitor how their resistance and motivation scores change over time (**Box 6**).

BRIEF MOTIVATIONAL INTERVENTIONS

Motivational interviewing (MI) is an evidence-based intervention for reducing problem drinking and other health risk behaviors[16] and has most recently been defined as "a

---

Box 5
Show the decision balance to the patient

Let me show you what a decision balance looks like. It can help you understand better your reasons to drink and your reasons to quit or cut down. (Pointing to the right upper quadrant), What do you like most about drinking alcohol? I will just make a note of what you say, so that you can keep a copy of it to look over.

Reproduced from Botelho RJ. Motivational practice: promoting healthy habits and self-care of chronic diseases. MHH Publications; 2004. Available at: www.MotivateHealthyHabits.com; with permission.

Table 7 Use decision balance		
Current Drinking Pattern	1. Benefits "What do you like about drinking alcohol?"	2. Concerns "Do you have any concerns about how alcohol affects your life?"
Low-Risk Drinking Limits or Abstinence	3. Concerns "What concerns would you have if you were to cut down to low-risk drinking limits (or abstain)?"	4. Benefits "What do you see as the benefits of cutting down to low-risk drinking limits (or abstaining)?

Reproduced from Botelho RJ. Motivational practice: promoting healthy habits and self-care of chronic diseases. MHH Publications; 2004; with permission.

collaborative, person-centered form of guiding to elicit and strengthen motivation for change."[17] This approach can be used alone or combined with other approaches, techniques, or assessment instruments.

The acronym OARS describes the techniques of MI: open-ended questions, affirmations, reflections, and summaries. To be effective, practitioners must deliver these techniques using the spirit of MI, which may involve evocation, collaboration, autonomy-supportiveness, empathy, and directiveness.[16] Evocation involves exploring patients' ambivalence about the target behavior with a concerted emphasis on their own thoughts, feelings, and beliefs in favor of change (ie, change talk). Collaboration suggests a joint decision-making process in which the practitioner's expert, authoritative position is often a barrier. Honoring and supporting patient autonomy requires the practitioner to truly accept and put faith into patients' wisdom to decide what, if any, change to make. As such, practitioners often must contain their desire to elicit immediate commitment from the patient to change the target behavior (ie, the righting reflex). The goal of an encounter may instead shift to taking some other step (eg, a follow-up appointment or referral). In addition, practitioner empathy presupposes a nonjudgmental, accepting, and warm attitude toward the patient and remains at the heart of this approach.

Recent studies have identified that the patient's change talk within a session can predict outcomes. The practitioner seeks to elicit and strengthen patient desire, ability,

Box 6 Explaining and obtaining resistance and motivation scores
The left column represents your reasons to drink (resistance). The right column represents your reasons to cut down or quit drinking (motivation). On a scale of 0 to 10, 0 meaning none and 10 meaning very high, what score would you give for your reasons to stay the same? (pointing to the left column) And what score would you give for your reasons to change? Are your resistance and motivation scores based on what you think or feel about change? Now how would you score your resistance and motivation based on what you feel (if a think score was given) or think (if a feeling score was given)?
Decision balances can help patients clarify and work their ambivalence about change. To watch a video of how to use a decision balance, go to www.MotivateHealthyHabits.com.
Reproduced from Botelho RJ. Motivational practice: promoting healthy habits and self-care of chronic diseases. MHH Publications; 2004. Available at: www.MotivateHealthyHabits.com; with permission.

reasons, need, and, ultimately, commitment (DARN-C) to change the health risk behavior. Paradoxically, accepting patient ambivalence about change encourages them to become increasingly forthcoming and express change talk instead of reacting to potential perceived threats to their freedom.[16,18]

To help patients abstain from drinking or reduce their alcohol intake, practitioners can use a blend of brief motivational interventions to help patients lower their resistance and increase their motivation (**Boxes 7** and **8**).[19] Brief video demonstrations of these interventions are available at: https://webmeeting.nih.gov/tutorial/.

REFERRAL TO TREATMENTS: INVOLVING FAMILY MEMBERS

Concerned significant others (CSOs) often encourage patients to accept referrals for assessments and possible treatment. In addition, programs such as community reinforcement and family training for CSOs can effectively engage two-thirds of substance abusers into treatment, who initially refused referrals.[20] Al-Anon is another useful support group for helping CSOs address their personal issues in relating to at-risk patients. (See Web-based resources for patients AUDIT score less than 7). Before referrals, practitioners can also ask at-risk patients to bring CSOs to support the therapy process.

REFERRAL PROCESS

Patients with substance-related health conditions or suspected substance use disorders warrant a formal diagnostic assessment and possible referral to treatment beyond a brief intervention.[21] About 50% to 65% of hospital patients identified with

---

Box 7
Nondirect interventions to lower patient resistance

Use simple reflections: "So drinking helps you to relax and sleep at night." "So sometimes your family gets upset with you." "You believe you have a right to do as you please in your own home."

Probe priorities to change: So, what is the most important reason for you to stay the same? And what is the most important reason for you to change?

Use double-sided reflection to explore ambivalence: On one hand, drinking alcohol helps you relax, but, on the other hand, your family gets upset with you.

Explore the future: So, what do you think your health will be like in 5 to 10 years if you carry on drinking alcohol at the same or higher levels?

Acknowledge ambivalence to validate patients' experience: So, it seems that you have mixed feelings about whether to continue or cut down on your drinking.

Emphasize personal responsibility and choice (useful when patients are being resistant): What you decide to do about drinking is entirely up to you. It's up to you to decide whether to change. You are the best judge of what will work for you. I'm here to help you explore your options and to support you in any way that will help you improve your health. That's what I see as my role.

Reproduced from Botelho RJ. Motivational practice: promoting healthy habits and self-care of chronic diseases. MHH Publications; 2004. Available at: www.MotivateHealthyHabits.com; with permission.

Box 8
Direct interventions to enhance patient motivation

Use back-to-the-future questioning

If you were to develop a health problem from your drinking now, would you stop drinking? (Provided that the patient shows some interest in prevention, continue with…) At the moment, you are drinking over the low-risk drink limit, which puts you at risk for developing complications. What do you think about that? (Alternative)

(If the patient remains interested in prevention…) What would it take for you to decide to drink alcohol below the low-risk limits? (If the patient is ambivalent or not interested in prevention…) (Study the patient's response/affect and offer a reflection) You are not too convinced that you are actually at risk."

Use benefit substitution

What other ways do you use to relax and deal with stress that does not involve drinking alcohol?

Identify discrepancies

"You love your partner, but he won't be with you if you drink." "You enjoy drinking with your friends for a while, but then you pay for it at home."

Use discrepancies

(In response to patient account of sleep apnea) Alcohol can help you fall asleep, but it gives you poor-quality sleep.

Provide information

Would you like to hear a bit about how that works? Alcohol makes you wake up during the night without you knowing it and reduces the amount of deep sleep that your body needs to give you more energy. In other words, you get poor-quality sleep, so you get tired more easily. So in the evening, when you have difficulties getting to sleep, you have a few drinks to fall asleep. This is a vicious cycle. You drink alcohol to fall sleep but get poor-quality sleep. What makes this more difficult is that when your body has become accustomed to the alcohol, you experience worse sleep problems when you stop drinking because of the rebound effect. It may take a week or so, sometimes longer, for your body to get over the effects of alcohol. It is quite complicated to understand how alcohol affects sleep. What do you think is the best way for you to improve your sleep and regain your energy so that you feel better?

Clarify values

What is more important, drinking to relax or sleeping better and having more energy for life?

Reframe events and issues

(Reflect in response to client statement that his partner "nags" about his drinking) She worries about you and is concerned about your health.

Use differences in motivational reasons

(In response to patient statement that work is unaffected and skepticism about the health consequences of at-risk or hazardous drinking) Your drinking has had no apparent effect on your performance at work, but it is difficult to know precisely what impact it is having on your health. You are very committed to doing a good job at work, but what would it take for you to do an even better job of taking care of your health in terms of reducing your alcohol intake to below low-risk limits?

Reproduced from Botelho RJ. Motivational practice: promoting healthy habits and self-care of chronic diseases. MHH Publications; 2004. Available at: www.MotivateHealthyHabits.com; with permission.

Box 9
Four levels of care
Level I is outpatient treatment, totaling fewer than 9 contact hours per week, and involves a combination of individual, family, and group therapy, as well as possible participation in support groups.
Level II is intensive outpatient treatment, including partial hospitalization, and provides a full array of treatment program exceeding 9 hours per week. Patients live at home or in special residences.
Level III is medically monitored intensive inpatient treatment. This level of care involves 24-hour observation, monitoring, and treatment. A multidisciplinary staff functions under medical supervision.
Level IV is medically managed intensive inpatient treatment; addiction professionals and clinicians provide a planned regimen of 24-hour medically directed evaluation, care, and treatment in an acute care inpatient setting. Patients generally have severe withdrawal or medical, emotional, or behavioral problems.
A list of recommended Web-based resources (http://www.myhq.com/public/s/b/sbirt/) for practitioners and patients can help health care organizations and practice settings implement SBIRT programs.

substance dependence during a screening process were effectively referred to specialized treatment as compared with 5% of control participants.[21]

Many factors affect the rates of substance abuse screening and treatment referrals. These factors include time, access to treatment, and financial issues for patients as well as reimbursement from third party payers.[22] Stigmatizing attitudes toward alcoholics and drug addicts, physicians' lack of knowledge about substance dependence, and their lack of self-efficacy in managing these problems inhibit effective patient referrals to treatment options.

Primary care teams need adequate reimbursement, organizational resources, and training to implement SBIRT as well as referral networks to match patient needs according to their level of care. Training in motivational interviewing can help practitioners work with and refer patients more effectively, even in brief encounters. Nurses, social workers, peer counselors, and other team members can provide more intensive follow-up services, such as brief strengths-based case management, which increase the engagement rate into treatment following referrals (Rapp and colleagues, 2008).[23]

REFERRAL OPTIONS

The American Society of Addiction Medicine's levels of care (**Box 9**) involve a spectrum of settings, treatment intensities, and types of delivery methods.[24]

APPENDIX 1: BRIEF ADVICE INTERVENTIONS

Introduction to brief interventions. Video: Helping Patients Who Drink Too Much. https://webmeeting.nih.gov/tutorial/

Case 1. Step 1: Ask about alcohol use
    https://webmeeting.nih.gov/case1/(Slides 1–8)

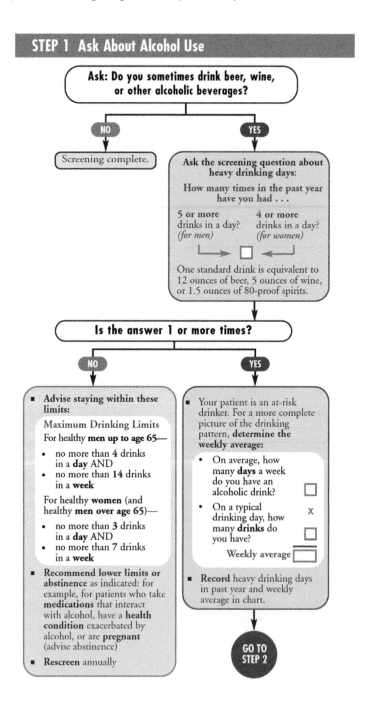

Case 1. Step 2: Assess for alcohol use disorders
https://webmeeting.nih.gov/case1/(Slides 9 and 10)

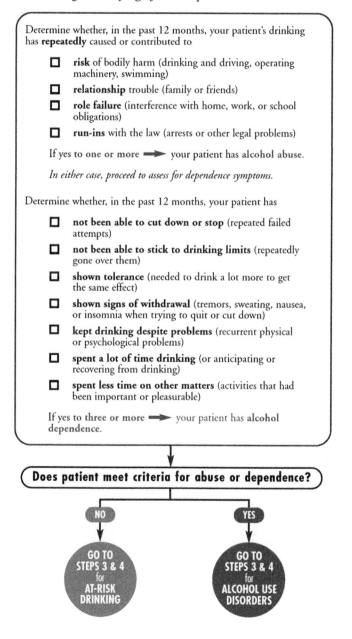

STEP 2 Assess For Alcohol Use Disorders

Next, determine if there is a *maladaptive pattern of alcohol use*, causing *clinically significant impairment* or *distress*.

Determine whether, in the past 12 months, your patient's drinking has **repeatedly** caused or contributed to

☐ **risk** of bodily harm (drinking and driving, operating machinery, swimming)

☐ **relationship** trouble (family or friends)

☐ **role failure** (interference with home, work, or school obligations)

☐ **run-ins** with the law (arrests or other legal problems)

If yes to one or more ➡ your patient has **alcohol abuse.**

In either case, proceed to assess for dependence symptoms.

Determine whether, in the past 12 months, your patient has

☐ **not been able to cut down or stop** (repeated failed attempts)

☐ **not been able to stick to drinking limits** (repeatedly gone over them)

☐ **shown tolerance** (needed to drink a lot more to get the same effect)

☐ **shown signs of withdrawal** (tremors, sweating, nausea, or insomnia when trying to quit or cut down)

☐ **kept drinking despite problems** (recurrent physical or psychological problems)

☐ **spent a lot of time drinking** (or anticipating or recovering from drinking)

☐ **spent less time on other matters** (activities that had been important or pleasurable)

If yes to three or more ➡ your patient has **alcohol dependence.**

Does patient meet criteria for abuse or dependence?

NO

YES

GO TO
STEPS 3 & 4
for
AT-RISK
DRINKING

GO TO
STEPS 3 & 4
for
ALCOHOL USE
DISORDERS

Case 1. Steps 3 and 4: Advice and assist (no abuse or dependence)
https://webmeeting.nih.gov/case1/ (Slides 11–22)

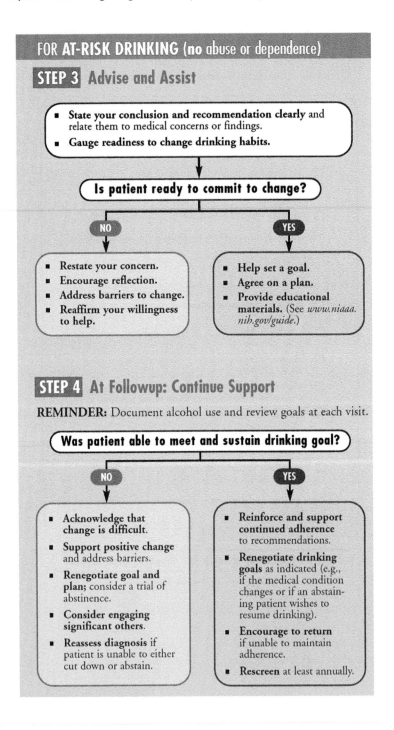

Case 1. Steps 3 and 4: Advice and assist (abuse or dependence)
https://webmeeting.nih.gov/case3/
https://webmeeting.nih.gov/case4/

FOR ALCOHOL USE DISORDERS (abuse or dependence)

STEP 3 Advise and Assist

- **State your conclusion and recommendation clearly** and relate them to medical concerns or findings.
- **Negotiate a drinking goal.**
- **Consider evaluation by an addiction specialist.**
- **Consider recommending a mutual help group.**
- For patients who have dependence, **consider**
  - the need for **medically managed withdrawal** (detoxification) and treat accordingly.
  - prescribing a **medication** for alcohol dependence for patients who endorse abstinence as a goal.
- **Arrange followup appointments**, including medication management support if needed.

STEP 4 At Followup: Continue Support

REMINDER: Document alcohol use and review goals at each visit.

Was patient able to meet and sustain drinking goal?

NO

- **Acknowledge that change is difficult.**
- **Support efforts** to cut down or abstain.
- **Relate drinking to ongoing problems** as appropriate.
- **Consider** (if not yet done):
  - consulting with an **addiction specialist.**
  - recommending a **mutual help group.**
  - engaging **significant others**.
  - prescribing a **medication** for alcohol-dependent patients who endorse abstinence as a goal.
- **Address coexisting disorders**—medical and psychiatric—as needed.

YES

- **Reinforce and support continued adherence.**
- **Coordinate care** with specialists as appropriate.
- **Maintain medications** for alcohol dependence for at least 3 months and as clinically indicated thereafter.
- **Treat coexisting nicotine dependence.**
- **Address coexisting disorders**—medical and psychiatric—as needed.

REFERENCES

1. U.S. Preventive Services Task Force. Screening and behavioral counseling interventions in primary care to reduce alcohol misuse: recommendation statement. Ann Intern Med 2004;140(7):554–6.
2. Bertholet N, Daeppen JB, Wietlisbach V, et al. Reduction of alcohol consumption by brief alcohol intervention in primary care: systematic review and meta-analysis. Arch Intern Med 2005;165(9):986–95.
3. Kaner EF, Beyer F, Dickinson HO, et al. Effectiveness of brief alcohol interventions in primary care populations. Cochrane Database Syst Rev 2007;2: CD004148.
4. Kaner EF, Dickinson HO, Beyer F, et al. The effectiveness of brief alcohol interventions in primary care settings: a systematic review. Drug Alcohol Rev 2009;28(3): 301–23.
5. Saitz R. Screening and brief intervention enter their 5th decade. Subst Abus 2007;28(3):3–6.
6. Bernstein E, Bernstein J, Feldman J, et al. An evidence-based alcohol screening, brief intervention and referral to treatment (SBIRT) curriculum for emergency department (ED) providers improves skills and utilization. Subst Abus 2007; 28(4):79–92.
7. McQueen J, Howe TE, Allan L, et al. Brief interventions for heavy alcohol users admitted to general hospital wards. Cochrane Database Syst Rev 2009; 3:CD005191.
8. Available at: http://www.nap.edu/openbook.php?record_id=1341. Accessed November 23, 2010.
9. Skinner HA. Spectrum of drinkers and intervention opportunities. CMAJ 1990; 143(10):1054–9.
10. Archer L, Grant BF, Dawson DA. What if Americans drank less? The potential effect on the prevalence of alcohol abuse and dependence. Am J Public Health 1995;85(1):61–6.
11. Kreitman N. Alcohol consumption and the preventive paradox. Br J Addict 1986; 81(3):353–63.
12. Saunders JB, Aasland OG, Babor TF, et al. Development of the alcohol use disorders identification test (AUDIT): WHO collaborative project on early detection of persons with harmful alcohol consumption–II. Addiction 1993;88(6): 791–804.
13. Ewing JA. Detecting alcoholism. The CAGE questionnaire. JAMA 1984;252(14): 1905–7.
14. Bush K, Kivlahan DR, McDonell MB, et al. The AUDIT alcohol consumption questions (AUDIT-C): an effective brief screening test for problem drinking. Ambulatory care quality improvement project (ACQUIP). Alcohol use disorders identification test. Arch Intern Med 1998;158(16):1789–95.
15. Reich T, Edenberg HJ, Goate A, et al. Genome-wide search for genes affecting the risk for alcohol dependence. Am J Med Genet 1998;81(3):207–15.
16. Rollnick S, Miller WR, Butler CC. Motivational interviewing in health care: helping patients change behavior. New York: Guilford Press; 2008.
17. Miller WR, Rollnick S. Ten things that motivational interviewing is not. Behav Cogn Psychother 2009;37(2):129–40.
18. Miller WR, Rollnick S. Motivational interviewing: preparing people for change. 2nd edition. New York: Guilford Press; 2002.

19. Botelho RJ. Motivational practice: promoting healthy habits and self-care of chronic diseases. MHH Publications; 2004. Available at: www.MotivateHealthyHabits.com. Accessed November 23, 2010.
20. Meyers RJ, Miller WR, Smith JE, et al. A randomized trial of two methods for engaging treatment-refusing drug users through concerned significant others. J Consult Clin Psychol 2002;70(5):1182–5.
21. Babor TF, McRee BG, Kassebaum PA, et al. Screening, brief intervention, and referral to treatment (SBIRT): toward a public health approach to the management of substance abuse. Subst Abus 2007;28(3):7–30.
22. Holland CL, Pringle JL, Barbetti V. Identification of physician barriers to the application of screening and brief intervention for problem alcohol and drug use. Alcohol Treat Q 2009;27(2):174–83.
23. Rapp RC, Otto AL, Lane DT, et al. Improving linkage with substance abuse treatment using brief case management and motivational interviewing. Drug Alcohol Depend 2008;94:172–82.
24. Hoffmann NG, Halikas JA, Mee-Lee D, et al. Patient placement criteria for the treatment of psychoactive substance use disorders (PPC-1). Washington, DC: American Society of Addiction Medicine; 1991.

Addiction Treatment: Level of Care Determination

Danesh A. Alam, MD[a,b,c,]*, Andrew Martorana, MD[a]

KEYWORDS

- Substance use • Addiction • Primary care • Level of care
- Appropriate referral

Substance use disorders occur in 10% to 20% of patients presenting to the primary care physician. Rates of illicit and prescription drug use are also increasing and may be in the range of 5% to 10% of all patients in primary care clinics. It is estimated that every fifth patient in a primary care practice has a substance use disorder. One in 5 inpatient admissions may be related to a substance use disorder.

Substance use disorders occur in approximately 10% to 15% of the adult population and contribute to significant costs to the society through lost productivity and excessive health care utilization.[1] Many studies in various settings, such as emergency rooms, general medical care, and psychiatric clinics, have reported that less than 15% of those who meet diagnostic criteria for a substance use disorder are referred to addiction treatment.[2] Of those that enter treatment, most drop out prematurely or receive an inadequate treatment. Predictably, this inadequate treatment leads to high premature dropout rates and relapse rates.

Alcoholism, more specifically, heavy drinking, is the third leading preventable cause of death in the United States, after smoking and obesity/lack of exercise.[3] According to one estimate, 54% of premature deaths due to alcohol consumption are because of acute conditions and 46% are because of chronic conditions.[4,5] Undoubtedly, alcohol use disorders are one of the most prevalent and expensive illnesses in health care. Current research evidence supports a significantly positive outcome in medical disorders if the substance use disorder is appropriately treated.

Significant advances have occurred in the treatment of chronic illnesses in primary care over the past 2 decades. Substance use disorders are considered chronic conditions. More recently, well-developed efforts have occurred to screen and intervene

The authors have nothing to disclose.
[a] Optum Health Behavioral Solutions, Suite 300, 1900 East Golf Road, Schaumburg, IL 60173, USA
[b] Central DuPage Hospital, 27 West 350 Highlake Road, Winfield, IL 60190, USA
[c] University of Illinois at Chicago, Chicago, IL, USA
* Corresponding author. Central DuPage Hospital, 27 West 350 Highlake Road, Winfield, IL 60190.
E-mail address: Danesh_Alam@cdh.org

Prim Care Clin Office Pract 38 (2011) 125–136
doi:10.1016/j.pop.2010.11.009
0095-4543/11/$ – see front matter © 2011 Elsevier Inc. All rights reserved.

primarycare.theclinics.com

early in chronic illnesses. Despite these efforts, there has been no meaningful increase in the rates of screening, early intervention, or referral to specialty care for addictive disorders among the general medical community.[6]

One of the challenges for the primary care physician after the initial assessment is a referral to the appropriate level of care. Substance abuse treatment is now a multibillion dollar industry, and there are a wide variety of options for those with resources. Most patients depend on community resources and state- and county-funded programs.

TREATMENT IN THE PRIMARY CARE OFFICE, INCLUDING SCREENING AND BRIEF INTERVENTIONS

For the primary care physician, the first step in approaching substance use disorders may be screening and brief intervention (SBI). This step is well studied and is generally applied to those individuals who are in the at-risk group and may not meet criteria for abuse or dependence. Monitoring and a referral to a higher level of care may be required if the substance use is not controlled. SBI are an important and well-researched approach to addressing addictive disorders. This intervention is delivered by the health care professional in the context of routine clinical care. It is essentially a focused session designed to reduce substance abuse. The average duration is 5 to 20 minutes. SBI works well with patients in all stages of motivation. The United States Preventive Services Task Force recommends routine SBI for problematic alcohol and tobacco use in primary care settings.[7] Screening may be done by using measures such as the CAGE (cut down, annoyed, guilty, eye opener) or AUDIT (Alcohol Use Disorders Identification Test) questionnaires. Several studies have demonstrated the effectiveness of the SBI in alcohol use. With SBI, alcohol use can be reduced by 10% to 30% during a 12-month period.[8]

Choosing an Appropriate Level of Care

Addiction treatment is often delivered separately from the medical/surgical delivery system. The insurance benefits for addiction treatment have been separate from health care benefits. The insurance coverage for addiction treatment may be much lower than medical/surgical benefit coverage. The recently passed Mental Health and Addiction Equity Act of 2008 is expected to change this.

Treatment settings vary widely with regard to services, especially with regard to medical services offered. The treatment philosophy may also vary. Assessment for treatment matching, knowledge of available treatment settings, and funding options in the community are important to make the appropriate referral. The continuum of care in addiction treatment facilitates the gradual movement from a more restrictive to a less restrictive level of care. Most programs provide an initial assessment with a specific level of care recommendations. Social work departments and managed care case managers may be able to provide assistance with local resources as well.

The following are factors that are considered in making this determination:

- Severity of illness and goals of treatment
- Comorbid conditions
- Relapse history
- Motivation
- Workplace risk
- Sober supports
- Resources, including insurance
- Local treatment resources.

As in other chronic illnesses, in addition to an initial intensive level of care, a plan for continuum of care may have to be considered to prevent relapses and maintain treatment-related gains.

Goals of Treatment

- Safe detoxification
- Address comorbid medical and psychiatric issues
- Motivational enhancement to facilitate treatment retention
- Skills to remain abstinent and prevent a relapse
- Offer a continuum of care to maintain treatment gains (**Table 1** and **Box 1**).

Placement of Patients in the Most Appropriate Treatment Setting

In the United States, only about 10% of substance use treatments are delivered in a 24 hour setting which includes inpatient and residential level of care.[9] The American Society of Addiction Medicine (ASAM) Patient Placement Criteria (PPC)[10,11] is probably the most-studied approach for matching the patient and treatment setting. The ASAM PPC criteria were first introduced in the 1980's and are now well accepted for patient placement. The ASAM PPC criteria provide guidelines for choosing the appropriate level of care. These criteria also help clinicians, third-party payers, and patients through facilitating the provision of individualized treatment. The criteria facilitated a movement away from fixed-length programs to clinically focused and outcome-oriented care.

About 30 US states require the use of at least some aspects of the ASAM criteria. Managed care also uses these criteria extensively for treatment authorization decisions. Ideally treatment decisions should not be influenced by insurance and reimbursement issues.

Assessment Dimensions

The ASAM criteria identify 6 assessment areas (dimensions) as the first step before making a patient placement decision. Refer to **Table 2**.

LEVELS OF CARE

The ASAM criteria conceptualize treatment in 5 basic levels of care:

- *Level 0.5*: early intervention (such as SBI)
- *Level I*: outpatient services
- *Level II*: intensive outpatient/partial hospitalization services
- *Level III*: residential/inpatient services
- *Level IV*: medically managed intensive inpatient services.

Choosing the Appropriate Level of Treatment

The ideal level of care is one that is least intensive, that addresses all the treatment needs, and that provides the individual the best opportunity to develop sobriety. Generally, a patient may begin treatment at a more intensive level and progress to a less intensive level of care.

Choosing the appropriate level of care is important. For example, a relapse may occur if a less intensive level of care than is appropriate is initiated.

Is there a consequence to choosing a more intensive level of care? There is no research evidence to the existence of a consequence to choosing a more intensive level of care than necessary. In the clinical experience of the authors, one debatable

Table 1
Principles of effective treatment

Serial No.	Principles	Remarks
1.	No single treatment is appropriate for all individuals	Matching treatment settings, interventions, and services to individuals' particular problems and needs is critical to their ultimate success in returning to productive functioning in the family, workplace and society
2.	Treatment needs to be readily available	Because individuals who are addicted to drugs may be uncertain about entering treatment, taking advantage of opportunities when they are ready for treatment is crucial. Potential treatment applicants can be lost if treatment is not immediately available or is not readily accessible
3.	Effective treatment attends to multiple needs of the individual	To be effective, treatment must address the individual's drug use and any associated medical, psychological, social, vocational, and legal problems
4.	An individual's treatment and services plan must be assessed continually and modified as necessary to ensure that the plan meets the person's changing needs	A patient may require varying combinations of services and treatment components during the course of treatment and recovery. In addition to counseling or psychotherapy, a patient at times may require medication, other medical services, family therapy, parenting instruction, vocational rehabilitation, and social and legal services. It is critical that the treatment approach be appropriate to the individual's age, gender, race/ethnicity, and culture
5.	Remaining in treatment for an adequate period is critical for treatment effectiveness	The appropriate duration for individuals depends on their problems and needs. Research indicates that, for most patients, the threshold of significant improvement is reached at about 3 mo in treatment. After this threshold is reached, additional treatment can produce further progress toward recovery. Because people often leave treatment prematurely, programs should include strategies to engage and keep patients in treatment
6.	Counseling (individual and group) and other behavioral therapies are critical components of effective treatment	In therapy, patients address issues of motivation, build skills to resist drug use, replace drug-using activities with constructive and rewarding nondrug-using activities and improve their problem-solving abilities. Behavioral therapy also facilitates interpersonal relationships and the individual's ability to function in the family and community
7.	Medications are an important element of treatment for many patients, especially when combined with counseling and other behavioral therapies	Methadone and ʟ-α-acetylmethadol are very effective in helping individuals addicted to heroin, and other opiates stabilize their lives and reduce their illicit drug use. Naltrexone is an effective medication for some opiate-dependent patients and some patients with co-occurring alcohol dependence. For persons addicted to nicotine, a nicotine replacement product (such as patches or gum) or an oral medication (such as bupropion) can be an effective component of treatment. For patients with co-occurring mental disorders, both behavioral treatments and medications, can be critically important

8.	Addicted or drug-abusing individuals with co-occurring mental disorders should have both disorders treated in an integrated way	Because addictive disorders and mental disorders often occur in the same individual, patients presenting for either condition should be assessed and treated for the co-occurrence of the other type of disorder
9.	Medical detoxification is only the first stage of addiction treatment and by itself does little to change long-term drug use	Medical detoxification safely manages the acute physical symptoms of withdrawal associated with stopping drug use. Although detoxification alone is rarely sufficient to help addicts achieve long-term abstinence, for some individuals it is a strongly indicated precursor to effective addiction treatment
10.	Treatment does not need to be voluntary to be effective	Strong motivation can facilitate the treatment process. Sanctions or enticements in the family, employment setting, or criminal justice system can significantly increase both entry into treatment and retention in treatment as well as the success of treatment interventions
11.	Possible drug use during treatment must be monitored continuously	Lapses to drug use can occur during treatment. The objective monitoring of a patient's drug and alcohol use during treatment, as through urinalysis or other tests, can help the patient withstand urges to use drugs. Such monitoring can also provide early evidence of drug use so that the individual's treatment plan can be adjusted. Feedback to patients who test positive for illicit drug use is an important element of monitoring
12.	Treatment programs should provide assessment for AIDS, hepatitis B and C, tuberculosis, and other infectious diseases and counseling to help patients modify or change behaviors that place themselves or others at risk for infection	Counseling can help patients avoid high-risk behaviors. Counseling can also help those who are already infected to manage their illnesses
13.	Recovery from drug addiction can be a long-term process and frequently requires multiple episodes of treatment. As with other chronic illnesses, relapses to drug use can occur during or after successful treatment episodes	Addicted individuals may require prolonged treatment and multiple episodes of treatment to achieve long-term abstinence and fully restore functioning. Participation in self-help support programs during and after treatment is often helpful in maintaining abstinence

Data from National Institute on Drug Abuse (1999). Principles of drug addiction treatment: a research-based guide. Rockville (MD): NIDA (NIH Publication No. 99-4180); 1999. p. 1–3.

Box 1
Components of comprehensive addiction treatment

Core Components of Addiction Treatment

    Intake processing/assessment

    Treatment planning

    Clinical and case management

    Substance use monitoring

    Behavioral therapy and counseling

    Pharmacotherapies

    Self-help/peer support groups

    Continuing care

Ancillary Services

    Mental health services

    Medical services

    HIV/AIDS services

    Educational services

    Vocational services

    Legal services

    Financial services

    Housing/transportation services

    Family services

    Child care services

The best treatment programs provide a combination of therapies and other services to meet the needs of the individual patient.

Abbreviation: HIV, human immunodeficiency virus.
Data from National Institute on Drug Abuse (1999). Principles of drug addiction treatment: a research-based guide. Rockville (MD): NIDA (NIH Publication No. 99-4180); 1999. p. 14.

---

reason for treatment noncompliance may be a referral to the most restrictive or highest level of care. When not indicated by the patient's individual needs.

Different Levels of Care

Detoxification

Detoxification is usually provided in a hospital setting. The goal of this procedure is stabilization of physical and emotional symptoms after a recent discontinuation of alcohol or other substances. The purpose of this stage is to prepare a patient to enter the rehabilitation stage of treatment (**Table 3**).

Detoxification can be provided at the following levels of care:

- Inpatient hospital based
- Residential
- Ambulatory.

This level of care is appropriate to address acute intoxication, severe medically complicated withdrawal, and co-occurring and medical or psychiatric conditions.

Table 2
The ASAM criteria assessment dimensions

Assessment Dimensions	Assessment and Treatment Planning Focus
1. Acute intoxication and/or withdrawal potential	Assessment for intoxication or withdrawal management. Detoxification in a variety of levels of care and preparation for continued addiction services
2. Biomedical conditions and complications	Assess and treat co-occurring physical health conditions or complications. Treatment provided within the level of care or through coordination of physical health services
3. Emotional, behavioral, or cognitive conditions and complications	Assess and treat co-occurring diagnostic or subdiagnostic mental health conditions or complications. Treatment provided within the level of care or through coordination of mental health services
4. Readiness to change	Assess stage of readiness to change. If not ready to commit to full recovery, engage into treatment using motivational enhancement strategies. If ready for recovery, consolidate and expand action for change
5. Relapse, continued use, or continued problem potential	Assess readiness for relapse prevention use or continued services and teach where problem potential is appropriate. Identify previous periods of sobriety or wellness and what worked to achieve this. If still at early stages of change, focus on raising consciousness of consequences of continued use or continued problems as part of motivational enhancement strategies
6. Recovery environment	Assess need for specific individualized family or significant other, housing, financial, vocational, educational, legal, transportation, and childcare services. Identify any supports and assets in any or all of the areas

Detoxification does not address the psychological, social, and behavioral problems associated with addiction and is analogous to a doorway, entry through which facilitates the initiation of recovery.

Hospital-based inpatient
Hospital-based inpatient level of care is the most restrictive and most expensive. This level of care is for patients who cannot otherwise be safely treated in a less-restrictive setting. This level of care is often provided in a primary psychiatric setting. In addition to addressing withdrawal-related complications, this level of care is appropriate for patients at a risk of suicide.

Residential programs, including therapeutic community
Residential programs provide care 24 hours a day, in nonhospital settings. Some are locked facilities but most are open voluntary treatment programs. Residential care is generally provided to patients who do not meet the clinical criteria for inpatient hospitalization but who are unable to maintain abstinence in an outpatient setting. Patients who are unlikely or unable to maintain abstinence may benefit from this highly structured setting.

There are regional and philosophic differences in the therapeutic approach. Most are fixed-length programs. Ideally, the duration of residential treatment should be determined by the clinical response to therapy, based on the ASAM PPC. Although there is evidence that some patients may benefit from programs of longer duration, patient willingness and resources may be barriers.

Table 3
The ASAM criteria levels of care

The ASAM PPC-2R Level of Detoxification Service for Adults	Level	Remarks
Ambulatory detoxification without extended onsite monitoring	I-D	Mild withdrawal with daily or less-than-daily outpatient supervision; likely to complete detoxification and to continue treatment or recovery
Ambulatory detoxification with extended onsite monitoring	II-D	Moderate withdrawal with all-day detoxification support and supervision; at night, has supportive family or living situation; likely to complete detoxification
Clinically managed residential detoxification	III.2-D	Minimal to moderate withdrawal, but needs 24-h support to complete detoxification and increase likelihood of continuing treatment or recovery
Medically monitored inpatient detoxification	III.7-D	Severe withdrawal and needs 24-h nursing care and physician visits as necessary; unlikely to complete detoxification without medical or nursing monitoring
Medically managed inpatient detoxification	IV-D	Severe, unstable withdrawal and needs 24-h nursing care and daily physician visits to modify detoxification regimen and manage medical instability
The ASAM PPC-2R levels of care	Level	Same levels of care for adolescents except Level III.3
Early intervention	0.5	Assessment and education for at-risk individuals who do not meet diagnostic criteria for substance-related disorder
Outpatient services	I	Less than 9 h of service per week (adults), less than 6 h/wk (adolescents) for recovery or motivational enhancement therapies/strategies
Intensive outpatient	II.1	9 h or more of service per week (adults), 6 h or more per week (adolescents) in a structured program to treat multidimensional instability
Partial hospitalization	II.5	20 h or more of service per week in a structured program for multidimensional instability not requiring 24-h care
Clinically managed low-intensity residential	III.1	24-h structure with available trained personnel with emphasis on reentry to the community; at least 5 h of clinical service per week
Clinically managed medium-intensity residential	III.3	24-h care with trained counselors to stabilize multidimensional imminent danger. Less intense milieu and group treatment for those with cognitive or other impairments unable to use full active milieu or therapeutic community

(continued on next page)

The ASAM PPC-2R Level of Detoxification Service for Adults	Level	Remarks
Table 3 *(continued)*		
Clinically managed high-intensity residential	III.5	24-h care with trained counselors to stabilize multidimensional imminent danger and prepare for outpatient treatment. Able to tolerate and use full active milieu or therapeutic community
Medically monitored intensive inpatient	III.7	24-h nursing care with physician availability for significant problems in dimensions 1, 2, or 3. 16-h/d counselor availability
Medically managed intensive inpatient	IV	24-h nursing care and daily physician care for severe unstable problems in dimensions 1, 2, or 3. Counseling available to engage patients in treatment
Opioid maintenance therapy	OMT	Daily or several times weekly opioid medication and counseling available to maintain multidimensional stability for those with opioid dependence

When the residential treatment model first emerged, it consisted of a 3- to 6-week inpatient phase followed by an extended outpatient phase with participation in self-help groups. The emergence of managed care led to a significant decline in lengths of stay.

Therapeutic community/transitional living programs
Therapeutic communities are one form of residential treatment, whereby the patient is expected to remain at this level of care for an extended period of time, usually from 6 to 12 months. Resocialization is probably the most important aspect of such programs. These programs are structured, and the individual is expected to demonstrate accountability, responsibility, and sobriety. Other residents also contribute to facilitating a peer support model.

The appropriate patient is one who has a history of chronicity and a history of multiple treatment failures. It is also common for individuals to be referred from the criminal justice system. The long-term outcome data for this level of care is somewhat limited. Data suggests that individuals who complete 12 to 24 months at this level of care are more likely to maintain long-term abstinence.

Community residential rehabilitation
Community residential rehabilitation facilities are also known as halfway houses or sober living communities. Patients appropriate for this setting are usually those who have a history of chronic relapses or those who are at a serious risk of relapse. Patients who are unemployed with few social supports may benefit from this environment. The barrier to referral to such programs is usually lack of patient motivation. Research supports a significant improvement in outcomes when this level of care is utilized.[12,13]

Clinical effectiveness of inpatient versus outpatient treatment
Addiction treatment is now a multibillion dollar business. Although considerable research efforts have attempted to focus on the benefits of inpatient versus outpatient level of care, it is still unclear if one level of care is more beneficial than the other.

The potential advantages of inpatient treatment are

- A safe environment facilitating the initiation of recovery
- Improved treatment retention, initially
- Availability of comprehensive medical and psychiatric services
- Better preparation for transition to outpatient treatment.

The advantages of outpatient treatment are

- Recovery in a real-world setting
- Cost-effectiveness
- Participation in 12-step groups in one's own community.

The initial research on comparative effectiveness of alcohol treatments concluded that inpatient or residential treatment was not more effective than outpatient treatment. Despite a large number of recent studies, significant methodological differences limit their usefulness.[14–16]

Smaller studies have noted an advantage of inpatient over outpatient treatments. A more important approach may be matching patients to the appropriate level of care. Patients in more advanced stages of addictive disease benefit from initial inpatient treatment. Patients with comorbid psychiatric disorders seem to benefit from residential treatment after having completed inpatient psychiatric treatment.[14] Patients with unemployment, poor family supports, and legal problems predictably had poorer outcomes in outpatient settings versus inpatient settings.

Patients with personality disorders had poorer outcomes in outpatient settings. With respect to the duration of treatment, current research suggests that there may be no benefit to long inpatient treatment, that is, programs with a duration longer than 15 months.[17] The length of stay in treatment programs is highly variable. A number of treatment programs have fixed length of stay.

Partial hospital programs

Partial hospitalization is an intermediate level of care for patients who require more intensive care than that provided by outpatient treatment. Partial hospitalization is also an outpatient level of care but is intensive and structured. It is often used as a continuum of care after an inpatient or residential treatment. In this level of care, treatment is provided daily for 6 to 8 hours. This level of care is appropriate for patients who are at a risk of relapse, who are returning to a high-risk environment, and who need to develop community supports. Patients with a lack of motivation, with comorbid psychiatric conditions, and with pain and addiction may benefit from this setting. This is the level of care that patients may be stepped up to for continued relapse behavior in an outpatient setting.

Partial hospital programs with boarding

Several partial hospital-based programs now offer a boarding component. The cost of boarding may not always be covered by insurance benefits and may be passed on to the patient if it is not reimbursable. This level of care allows more patients to reside in a controlled environment while in treatment. Some programs allow patients to continue to board when they enter the intensive outpatient program.

Intensive outpatient programs

The main difference between partial hospital programs and intensive outpatient is in the intensity, number of hours per day, setting of the program, and structure of the program. There is a significant variation in the intensity and structure nationwide. In general, treatment is provided for 3 to 5 hours, 3 to 6 times a week.

Outpatient programs
This is the least restrictive level of care and the ideal patient is one who

- Is in the early stages of addictive disease, with few or no complications
- Shows good insight
- Has good compliance
- Has resources and social supports.

A comprehensive approach with multiple modalities, such as psychotherapy, medication therapy, family therapy, and monitoring, predict better outcomes. In general, most alcohol abuse/dependence, cannabis abuse/dependence, cocaine abuse/dependence, and nicotine abuse or dependence are addressed at an outpatient level of care, barring the presence of other comorbidities.[18]

Good outcome is probably dependent on treatment retention.

AFTERCARE PROGRAMS

Most patients are referred to aftercare after completion of the primary treatment. Aftercare program usually consists of weekly group therapy with involvement in 12-step programs. The duration varies across programs but is generally expected to continue from 6 to 12 months.

CLINICAL MONITORING

One area of care that is not frequently used by primary care providers is the use of drug testing and monitoring of abstinence. As in other chronic illnesses, underreporting is common in addictive disorders.

When drug testing is done in addition to history taking, physical examination, and diagnosis, it can provide important clinical information. The clinicians' own discomfort about dealing directly with issues related to substance use disorders may sometimes be a barrier. Concerns about continued drug use should be addressed in a nonjudgmental and nonconfrontational manner, which predicts improved clinical outcomes in general and with other comorbid medical or psychiatric disorders.[19]

It is clear that more research is needed in guiding the primary care physician in an approach to managing addictive disorders. Meanwhile, what is a clinician to do?

The recent introduction of pharmacotherapeutic interventions, such as acamprosate calcium (Campral) and naltrexone (Vivitrol), has expanded the options available to the clinician. At present, only about 20% of eligible patients are offered this option.[20] One review has also noted that commercial insurance only covers about 10% of patients seeking treatment. The clinical approach to patients should be as with any chronic illness, all patients should be screened and referrals made as appropriate. The primary care physician is probably most influential in helping patients make appropriate decisions. The most appropriate level of care for a patient is one that addresses all the patient's needs and that reduces the risk of relapse and allows for initiation and maintenance of recovery. At this time, the data do not support inpatient treatment over outpatient treatment, and this decision has to be based on the needs of the patient. The ASAM placement criteria are a guide to placement decisions.

REFERENCES

1. Harwood HJ, Fountain D, Livermore G. The economic costs of alcohol and drug abuse in the United States. Rockville (MD): National Institute on Drug Abuse; 1998.

2. National Household Survey on Drug Use and Health (NHSDUH): results from the 2006 survey. SAMHSA. Available at: http://www.oas.samhsa.gov/nsduh. Accessed August 11, 2008.

3. Mokdad AH, Marks JS, Stroup DF, et al. Actual causes of death in the United States, 2000. JAMA 2004;291(10):1238–45.

4. Chikritzhs TN, Jonas HA, Stockwell TR, et al. Mortality and life-years lost due to alcohol: a comparison of acute and chronic causes. Med J Aust 2001;174(6): 281–4.

5. Willenbring ML. Medications to treat alcohol dependence: adding to the continuum of care. JAMA 2007;298(14):1691–2.

6. Bodenheimer T, Wagner E, Grumbach K. Improving primary care for patients with chronic illness. JAMA 2002;288(14):1775–9.

7. U.S. Preventive Services Task Force. Guide to clinical preventive services, 2007: recommendations. Available at: http://www.ahrq.gov/clinic/. Accessed January 23, 2008.

8. Whitlock EP, Polen MR, Green CA, et al, U.S. Preventive Services Task Force. Behavioral counseling interventions in primary care to reduce risky/harmful alcohol use by adults: a summary of the evidence for the U.S. Preventive Services Task Force. Ann Intern Med 2004;140:557–68.

9. Substance Abuse and Mental Health Services Administration, Office of Applied Studies National Survey of Substance Abuse Treatment (NSSAT): 2005. Data on substance abuse treatment facilities. Rockville (MD): (Vol. DHHS Publication No. SMA 06-4206); 2006.

10. Mee-Lee D, Shulman GD, Gartner L. ASAM patient placement criteria for the treatment of substance-related disorders. (ASAM PPC-2). 2nd edition. Chevy Chase (MD): American Society of Addiction Medicine; 1996.

11. Leukfeld C, Pickens R, Shuster CR. Improving drug abuse treatment recommendation for research and practice. Improving drug abuse treatment (NIDA research monograph series). Rockville (MD): NIDA; 1991.

12. Friedmann PD, Hendrickson JC, Gerstein DR, et al. The effect of matching comprehensive services to patients' needs on drug use improvement in addiction treatment. Addiction 2004;99:962–72.

13. DeLeon G, Scnhwartz S. Therapeutic communities: what are the retention rate? Am J Drug Alcohol Abuse 1984;10:267–84.

14. Moos RH, King M, Patterson M. Outcomes of residential treatment of substance abuse in hospital-versus community-based programs. Psychiatr Serv 1996;47: 68–74.

15. Finney JW, Moos RH. Effectiveness of inpatient and outpatient treatment for alcohol abuse: effect sizes, research design issues, and explanatory mechanisms [response to commentaries]. Addiction 1996;91:1813–20.

16. Miller MR, Hester RK. Inpatient alcoholism treatment: who benefits? Am Psychol 1986;41:794–805.

17. Mattick RP, Jarvis T. In-patient setting and long duration for the treatment of alcohol dependence? Out-patient care is as good. Drug Alcohol Rev 1994;13: 127–35.

18. Institute of Medicine. Treating drug problems. Washington, DC: National Academy Press; 1990.

19. Warner EA, Friedman PD. Laboratory testing for drug abuse. Arch Pediatr Adolesc Med 2006;160:854–64.

20. Alam D, Angres D. Advances in pharmacotherapy of alcoholism. Int Drug Ther Newsl 2007;42(3).

Primary Care of the Patient in Recovery

Robert Mallin, MD[a,b]

KEYWORDS

• Addiction • Insomnia • Relapse

It is not known what percentage of the greater than 20% of addicted primary care patients are in recovery from their disease. Although treatment centers frequently encourage patients to speak to their physicians about their recovery, many patients are reluctant to do so. The lack of familiarity many primary care doctors have with recovery reinforces this reluctance. In the long view, however, it is likely that the primary care physician will have more contact than other health care professionals with the patient in recovery and consequently needs to have a thorough understanding of the principles of recovery. The patients' personal physician can and should play a pivotal role in their recovery. Aside from knowledge of the principles of recovery, the most important factor in working with these patients may be the nature of the patient-physician relationship. The importance of a nonjudgmental, supportive relationship with the patient in recovery cannot be overstated. A solid understanding of the disease process and of recovery will be useless if the patient is lost secondary to poor interview skills. The physician should convey concern, respect, and empathy by using open-ended questions and active listening. Affirmation of the patients' successes will build the therapeutic relationship more effectively than advice giving. Patients in recovery from addiction have often had negative experiences with health care professionals and can be very sensitive to a judgmental or nonsupportive attitude.[1]

Often, if the patient has been to addiction treatment, an aftercare contract has been completed. Aftercare contracts generally are negotiated in treatment and spell out in great detail the tasks needed to prevent relapse. Frequently, they address issues such as frequency of attendance to 12-step recovery meetings, attendance in aftercare therapy groups, an agreement to begin and maintain a relationship with a sponsor, and drug screening in the workplace or aftercare site. Generally, they also include an agreement about who is to be informed of the patient's progress, and often they

[a] Family Medicine, Medical University of South Carolina, 295 Calhoun Street Room 126, Charleston, SC 29425, USA
[b] Psychiatry and Behavioral Science, Medical University of South Carolina, 295 Calhoun Street Room 126, Charleston, SC 29425, USA
E-mail address: mallinr@musc.edu

Prim Care Clin Office Pract 38 (2011) 137–142
doi:10.1016/j.pop.2010.12.001   primarycare.theclinics.com

include the need to name a primary care physician who can cooperate with this process. The importance of monitoring aftercare agreements can be supported by the fact that physicians in recovery from addiction who participate in a strict monitoring program have considerably better outcomes (73%–94%) than physicians who do not participate in monitoring (44%–68%).[2,3]

Box 1 gives a list of points to cover when considering the monitoring of patients in recovery from addiction. In a routine primary care visit, it is not reasonable to cover each of these points, but it should be possible to cover 1 or 2 in each visit, thereby covering the entire list over time.

ABSTINENCE

The cornerstone of recovery from addiction is abstinence. Strictly interpreted, abstinence implies that the patient is consuming no mood-altering substances except under the direction of a physician. It is the recovering person's responsibility to be sure that the physician who may be prescribing a mood-altering substance knows that the patient is in recovery and that he has some understanding of the disease of addiction and recovery. This concern should include over-the-counter medications and dietary supplements, which may have potential to result in relapse. The patient should be cautioned to avoid medications that may affect mood, contain alcohol, or those for which the effect may be unknown. The willingness with which patients turn over the decisions regarding medication to a negotiation with their physician can be a good indication of the quality of their recovery. The ability to maintain abstinence, or prevent relapse, is the primary task of a patient in recovery. The primary care physician can help in this task by monitoring the process by which it is accomplished. A straightforward question such as "Have you had any mood altering substances, either prescribed or otherwise since our last visit?" is appropriate. Some aftercare

---

Box 1
Recovery checklist

1. Abstinence: has the patient remained abstinent from all mood-altering substances since the last visit?

2. Meetings: what recovery group meeting is the patient attending? Frequency? Involvement? What step are they working on?

3. Sponsor: frequency of contact with sponsor?

4. Emotional symptoms: mood, anger, depression, guilt, anxiety, psychotherapy, medications, and compliance.

5. Physical health: health maintenance, medications, compliance.

6. Exercise: frequency? Type?

7. Leisure activities: frequency? Type?

8. Work: occupation, work schedule, satisfaction.

9. Financial issues: debt and so on.

10. Compulsive behavior: exercise, work, food, sex, gambling, spending.

11. Legal issues.

12. Family/Relationship issues.

13. Spiritual support.

contracts call for random urine drug screens, and for some patients this may be a useful tool. The primary care physician should negotiate an agreement with the patient that allows him to ask for a drug screen, should a question arise.

MEETING ATTENDANCE

Recent data support the concept that 12-step recovery can help prevent relapse.[4,5] The usual recommendation is for the patients to attend at least 90 meetings in the first 90 days of their recovery. Some steps down from this approach may be negotiated after the first 90 days, but the patient's sponsor ought to be involved in that negotiation. In addition to meeting attendance, involvement in the fellowship has been shown to be important. Some attention to this in monitoring is important. Is the patient making new relationships in the meetings? Are they getting involved in the setting up or breaking down process of the meeting? Are they doing service work, such as making coffee, helping other recovering persons, and chairing meetings? Some patients complain that they have difficulty connecting in 12-step recovery groups. Frequently, they complain of religious issues associated with their dislike of recovery groups. It is important to emphasize that these groups may be spiritual in nature but are not religious. Encourage the patient to try different groups to find one that is acceptable. Often contacting someone in alcoholics anonymous (AA) who has a similar occupation or background can help make the patient more comfortable.

SPONSOR CONTACT

Serious work in 12-step recovery requires a sponsor.[6] In treatment, patients are encouraged to find someone of the same sex, who has qualities they respect to ask to sponsor them. Often these relationships begin as temporary sponsor relationships and may become permanent. Frequent contact with one's sponsor is usually encouraged but is typically negotiated between the sponsor and the patient. Although some sponsors prefer to remain anonymous with regard to a patient's primary care physician, many are willing to work closely with the doctor to maximize the patient's chances to avoid relapse. An important question to ask a patient in early recovery is "What step are you and your sponsor working on?" A hesitant or vague response is often a red flag that should prompt further inquiry.

EMOTIONAL SYMPTOMS

Patients in early recovery often are dealing with newly discovered or rediscovered emotions. Fear, anger, guilt, and depression are emotional traps that can lead to relapse if not appropriately handled. Individual or group psychotherapy, treatment for comorbid psychiatric disorders, should all be monitored. Often the acronym HALT is used in 12-step recovery to refer to the fact that patients in early recovery should avoid getting too Hungry, Angry, Lonely, or Tired, lest they risk relapse.

PHYSICAL HEALTH

Patients with addiction often have neglected their physical health for long periods. They may be well behind on their health surveillance. In addition, evaluation for the possible medical consequences of addiction must be maintained. Patients in good recovery are likely to be vigilant about medication compliance, keeping appointments, and appropriate concern about their physical health. Changes in these areas may be a sign of impending relapse.[7]

EXERCISE

Patients in active addiction have rarely maintained an adequate exercise program. This is an area that should be monitored for compulsive use. Sometimes patients in recovery may exercise compulsively as a replacement for their compulsive drug use.[8]

LEISURE ACTIVITIES

Patients in active addiction frequently become isolated, spending more and more of their time engaged in drug use. They may have forgotten how to have fun in a sober way. Encouraging the patient to become involved in social activities with their 12-step recovery group is one way to promote healthy leisure activity. One should be circumspect about leisure activities in the presence of people who are using or abusing alcohol or other drugs, especially early in recovery.

WORK ISSUES

Consequences of addiction frequently involve work. There may be a monitoring program in the workplace, which involves the patient. Work is another area that compulsive behavior may be acted out and should be watched for.

FINANCIAL PROBLEMS

This is a well-known area for concern regarding relapse. As with work, there are often considerable financial consequences resulting from active addiction that must be addressed, often in early recovery. Encouraging the patient to seek professional assistance in this area and not get further behind is a good advice.

COMPULSIVE BEHAVIOR

The transfer of compulsive behavior from drugs to other behaviors is a well-known phenomenon in early recovery. Attention to issues such as compulsive eating, purging, exercise, work, gambling, and sex is important to head off these potential relapse traps.[9]

LEGAL ISSUES

Legal consequences may complicate early recovery. Again, professional assistance is desirable and should not be put off.

FAMILY AND RELATIONSHIP ISSUES

Often an ongoing area of conflict, family therapy is often recommended to deal with these issues that are potential relapse traps.

SPIRITUAL SUPPORT

Understanding that the heart of 12-step recovery is spiritual, the physician should encourage the patient to continue to pursue spiritual growth. Recognition that this is not the same as religious pursuits may be important to some patients.

Common Medical Problems in Recovery

Because of the risk of relapse, patients in recovery must often have their medical problems managed in a manner different than other patients.

Sleep Disorders

Insomnia is common, especially early in recovery, and may be a sign of withdrawal (especially from opiates or sedative hypnotics). Reassurance that a normal sleep pattern will return is often the only intervention necessary. Unfortunately, this is a slow process and may take months to resolve. Sleep hygiene education is often useful. Avoiding hypnotics, especially benzodiazepines, barbiturates, and zolpidem is appropriate. Tricyclic antidepressants are probably safe but are also best avoided unless depression is present.

Pain

The appropriate treatment of pain is an important part of caring for the individual in recovery. Inadequate treatment of pain has proved to be as risky as over prescribing in terms of relapse. Pain tolerance in recovering addicts may be reduced, and tolerance to analgesics may be increased, even after recovery. Following the usual approach of using less dangerous drugs such as acetaminophen and nonsteroidal antiinflammatory agents is appropriate. If these are ineffective, short-term use of narcotic analgesics is appropriate, dose adjusted to relieve pain, followed, if necessary by detoxification.[10] In general, the recovering addict may become physically dependent more quickly than other patients. Safety of the use of these agents may be improved by using sponsor or spouse to help provide accountability, agreement to adhere to strict dosing schedule, frequent monitoring, and increased attention to other areas of recovery. Long-term opiate use has been shown to be safe for the treatment of chronic benign pain in nonaddicted individuals. There is no evidence that it is safe in those in recovery for addiction. In general, where possible, avoidance of controlled substances in patients recovering from addiction is a good policy. If the patient is suffering from chronic pain, referral to a pain management specialist who understands addiction is important.

Anxiety disorders, common in early recovery, may be a sign of withdrawal. Avoidance of controlled substances (including clonazepam) is important. Behavioral approaches, buspirone, β-blockers, and selective serotonin uptake inhibitors may be useful and safe.[11]

Depression

A high comorbidity of depressive symptoms in early recovery may be in part secondary to a substance-induced mood disorder that will resolve with abstinence. Comorbid depression does occur however and should be addressed, because it can negatively affect outcome. Antidepressants seem to be safe in recovery, and psychotherapy is often effective.

Over-the-Counter and Prescription Medication Use

Any mood-altering substance has the potential to contribute to relapse. Patients need to know this and need to be encouraged to ask for the physician's guidance before using these substances. In general, self-prescribing should be discouraged, and there should be an agreement with the patient in recovery that the physician will be apprised of any other medications or supplements he or she is taking. Some addictive substances are currently not controlled. Some of the headache preparations that contain butalbital, Stadol nasal spray, and tramadol are not controlled but are known to have caused relapse.

REFERENCES

1. Friedmann PD, Saitz R, Samet JH. Management of adults recovering from alcohol or other drug problems. JAMA 1998;279(15):1227–31.
2. Talbott GD, Gallegos KV, Angres DH. Impairment and recovery in physicians and other helath professionals. In: Graham AW, Shultz TK, editors. Principles of addiction medicine. Second edition. Maryland: American Society of Addiction Medicine Chevy Chase; 1998. p. 1265–80.
3. Dupont RL, McLellan A, White WL, et al. Gold MS Setting the Standard for Recovery: Physicians' Health Programs. J Subst Abuse Treat 2009;36:159–71.
4. Project MATCH Research Group. Project MATCH secondary a priori hypotheses. Addiction 1997;92:1671–98.
5. Kaskutas Lee Ann, Ammon Lyndsay, Delucchi Kevin, et al. Alcoholics anonymous careers: patterns of AA involvement five years after treatment entry. Alcohol Clin Exp Res 2005;29(11):1983–90.
6. Humphreys K. Alcoholics Anonymous and 12-step alcoholism treatment programs. Recent Dev Alcohol 2003;16(III):149–64.
7. McLellan AT, Lewis DC, O'Brien CP, et al. Drug dependence, a chronic medical illness implications for treatment, insurance, and outcomes evaluation. JAMA 2000;284:1689–95.
8. Read JP, Brown RA, Marcus BH, et al. Exercise attitudes and behaviors among persons in treatment for alcohol use disorders. J Subst Abuse Treat 2001; 21(4):199–206.
9. Tavares H, Zilberman ML, Hodgins DC, et al. Comparison of craving between pathological gamblers and alcoholics. Alcohol Clin Exp Res 2005;29(8):1427–31.
10. Weaver M, Schnoll S. Abuse liability in opioid therapy for pain treatment in patients with an addiction history. Clin J Pain 2002;18(4):S61–9.
11. Brady KT, Tolliver BK, Verduin ML. Alcohol use and anxiety: diagnostic and management issues. Am J Psychiatry 2007;164:217–21.

Alcoholics Anonymous and Other Twelve-Step Programs in Recovery

D. Todd Detar, DO

KEYWORDS

• Alcoholics Anonymous • Twelve Steps
• Abstinence • Recovery

Today, millions of people are in "recovery," living life because of the Twelve-Step programs of recovery. There are recovery groups for everything from alcohol to weight problems covering the globe. The Alcoholics Anonymous (AA) was started in 1935 by 2 men Bill W and Dr Bob who experienced relief from alcohol consumption by talking and being with each other. Bill W convinced Dr Bob of the similarities of the disease model of alcoholism, thus providing a foundation for the sobriety of both men and the beginning of a new change in life, which neither man had known.

The Twelve Steps of AA are the foundation of the AA, describing both the necessary actions and the spiritual basis for the recovery program of AA. The Twelve Steps of AA provide a structure for which a patient with alcoholism may turn for an answer to their problem of alcohol use, abuse, or dependence (**Fig. 1**).

The Twelve Traditions of AA are the guidelines for AA groups to survive conflict and function smoothly without a structured organization (**Fig. 2**).

The AA members enter groups by several routes, including physician referrals. In one study, examining data from the National Health Interview Survey of 43,809 adults in the United States, 5.8% adults had attended AA at some point in their lives.[1] Data from the National Epidemiological Survey on Alcohol and Related Conditions[2] reported a 20.1% attendance rate in respondents with a history of alcohol dependence.[3] Several cross-sectional and longitudinal studies suggest different patterns of use of the AA meetings.[4–6] Research reveals that not only attendance but also involvement in the AA group is associated with higher abstinence rates and improved outcomes.[7,8]

There is resistance to attending AA from patients. The reasons are diverse and numbered. Typically, physicians encounter patients who are atheists, agnostics, or of

Department of Family Medicine, Medical University of South Carolina, 295 Calhoun Street, Charleston, SC 29425, USA
E-mail address: detardt@musc.edu

Prim Care Clin Office Pract 38 (2011) 143–148
doi:10.1016/j.pop.2010.12.002
0095-4543/11/$ – see front matter © 2011 Elsevier Inc. All rights reserved.

Service Material from the General Service Office

THE TWELVE STEPS OF ALCOHOLICS ANONYMOUS

1. We admitted we were powerless over alcohol—that our lives had become unmanageable.

2. Came to believe that a Power greater than ourselves could restore us to sanity.

3. Made a decision to turn our will and our lives over to the care of God *as we understood Him.*

4. Made a searching and fearless moral inventory of ourselves.

5. Admitted to God, to ourselves, and to another human being the exact nature of our wrongs.

6. Were entirely ready to have God remove all these defects of character.

7. Humbly asked Him to remove our shortcomings.

8. Made a list of all persons we had harmed, and became willing to make amends to them all.

9. Made direct amends to such people wherever possible, except when to do so would injure them or others.

10. Continued to take personal inventory and when we were wrong promptly admitted it.

11. Sought through prayer and meditation to improve our conscious contact with God, *as we understood Him*, praying only for knowledge of His will for us and the power to carry that out.

12. Having had a spiritual awakening as the result of these Steps, we tried to carry this message to alcoholics, and to practice these principles in all our affairs.

Rev. 5/9/02

Fig. 1. The Twelve Steps of AA. (Copyright © Alcoholics Anonymous World Services, Inc.)

different religious perspective; because of the resistance or other reasons not explained, professionals are less likely to refer these patients to a Twelve-Step program in these cases. When professionals do refer patients and encourage patients to attend an AA group, attendance was positively associated with improved outcomes regardless of religious beliefs.[9,10] Comorbid psychiatric illnesses were also studied. Bogenschutz[11] noted that when patients with comorbid psychiatric disorders attended the AA at the same rate as other patients, patients with comorbid psychiatric problems did better in specialized groups for the associated disorder.[11-13]

Service Material from the General Service Office

THE TWELVE TRADITIONS OF ALCOHOLICS ANONYMOUS

(SHORT FORM)

1. Our common welfare should come first; personal recovery depends upon A.A. unity.

2. For our group purpose there is but one ultimate authority—a loving God as He may express Himself in our group conscience. Our leaders are but trusted servants; they do not govern.

3. The only requirement for A.A. membership is a desire to stop drinking.

4. Each group should be autonomous except in matters affecting other groups or A.A. as a whole.

5. Each group has but one primary purpose—to carry its message to the alcoholic who still suffers.

6. An A.A. group ought never endorse, finance, or lend the A.A. name to any related facility or outside enterprise, lest problems of money, property, and prestige divert us from our primary purpose.

7. Every A.A. group ought to be fully self-supporting, declining outside contributions.

8. Alcoholics Anonymous should remain forever nonprofessional, but our service centers may employ special workers.

9. A.A., as such, ought never be organized; but we may create service boards or committees directly responsible to those they serve.

10. Alcoholics Anonymous has no opinion on outside issues; hence the A.A. name ought never be drawn into public controversy.

11. Our public relations policy is based on attraction rather than promotion; we need always maintain personal anonymity at the level of press, radio, and films.

12. Anonymity is the spiritual foundation of all our Traditions, ever reminding us to place principles before personalities.

Rev.5/9/02

Fig. 2. The Twelve Traditions of AA. (Copyright © Alcoholics Anonymous World Services, Inc.)

Studies have researched the contribution of the AA attendance and involvement to predict successful resolution of an alcohol problem. Positive outcomes, including abstinence at 5-, 8-, and 16-years follow-ups, are related to the AA attendance and involvement as seen in treatment populations in the 1990s compared with patients not attending the AA groups.[14–16] A 5-year follow-up study by Gossop and colleagues[17] found a positive association between the AA/Narcotics Anonymous attendance and abstinence from opiates and alcohol but not from stimulants. Studies comparing patients who attended treatment centers alone without the AA and patients who attended the AA groups alone showed similar results, with patients involved in a treatment program, whether inpatient or extensive outpatient, and the AA groups being almost twice as likely to have successful outcomes as those involved with formal treatment alone.[3,16,18,19]

With the evidence that AA is beneficial for many problems, drinkers researchers are now looking at the mechanism of change and why it is beneficial. First, investigators are looking at what ingredients cause the change. Second, these ingredients must produce change that enhances the probability of successful behavior changes, and third, these changes in an individual must predict later reductions in drinking.

Emrick[20] described the meeting attendance as the "dose" and frequency of meeting attendance as the intensity of the dose. Montgomery and colleagues[21] distinguished between attendance and involvement-included participation during meetings, having a sponsor, leading meetings, working the Twelve Steps, and doing the Twelve-Step work. Involvement and attendance were moderately correlated with lower posttreatment consumption. However, involvement, not attendance, correlated with lower posttreatment consumption in a sample of patients in an inpatient Twelve-Step treatment program. Involvement is an active process as opposed to passively attending meetings. Tonigan[22] used the Project MATCH data to examine the nature of the participants' experience with the AA. Greater participation was reflected in a combination of the following factors: (1) a spiritual awakening, (2) God consciousness, (3) the perception that attending the AA meetings was helpful, (4) attending the AA meetings, (5) being involved in the AA-related practices, and (6) completing more steps. Participation in the AA during treatment and in the first 6 months after treatment predicted better drinking outcomes in the second 6 months after treatment.[22] Several AA-related behaviors for abstinence reported by the AA members were confirmed by Pagano and colleagues.[23] The investigators reexamined the Project MATCH data set and reported that being an AA sponsor led to a significant reduction in relapse rate at 1 year (60% vs 78%). Witbrodt and Kaskutas[24] investigated whether the type of substance use disorder (ie, alcohol dependence, drug dependence, or both) moderated the relative benefits of the Twelve-Step meeting attendance and prescribed behaviors. The investigators found that of the 7 specific AA behaviors, only having a sponsor predicted positive outcomes across substance abuse categories. Research has been done to look at other behaviors in the AA fellowship. The number of steps completed at 3-years follow-up and alcohol consumed at 10-years follow-up was significantly and negatively related. Also, commitment to and understanding of the Twelve Steps were significantly and positively predictive at 1-year abstinence.[2,15]

The social variables have also been studied with variable outcomes. Patients with networks made up of the Twelve-Step members had a higher quality of friendship than networks made up of almost no Twelve-Step members.[25] Social networks supportive of abstinence with the Twelve-Step programs may vary temporally. Alcohol-dependent patients with the Twelve-Step network support for abstinence were predictive of abstinence at 6-months follow-up but not at 12-months follow-up. With narcotic-dependent patients, the reverse was observed at 6 months, but abstinence was improved at 12 months.[24] This phenomenon may be related to unintended triggers during early efforts to remain abstinent. The Twelve-Step facilitation treatment centers improve social networks, which predict improved abstinence.

The Twelve-Step programs are not for everyone. Atheists and agnostics tend to not participate in these programs, but those who participate have higher abstinent rates at 6 and 12 months.[26] If individuals seek the program voluntarily, a substantial portion turn to the AA as sole assistance, or with formal treatment, many individuals who are self-seekers or have been coerced to come are very likely to continue their involvement for many years if they stay with AA for more than a year. This involvement is clearly correlated with positive outcomes in terms of reduced drinking, improved psychological functioning, and better social support systems.

Physicians can encourage patients to find an AA meeting where they may feel comfortable or find similarities with the group. Physicians must advocate that these patients find a sponsor or mentor to guide them through the Twelve Steps, to attend meetings, to become involved with the group, and to become a sponsor; overall, the more active patients become in the AA, the better the outcomes.

Assessment of recovery also mirrors our advocacy. Do you go to meetings? Do you have a sponsor? How involved are you with the AA? Are you willing to talk about your problem? When was your last drink? These questions allow us to further look into the life of alcoholic patients or addicts and their program of recovery.

Recovery is a new way of life for many of these patients; a life without substances to alter their moods but with a major change improving the physical, psychological, and emotional stability with improved overall health outcomes. The AA neither charges a fee for attendance nor advertises. Increased methodological sophistication and creativity in research in the AA is ongoing.

REFERENCES

1. Hasin DS, Grant BF. AA and other helpseeking for alcohol problems: former drinkers in the U.S. general population. J Subst Abuse 1995;7(3):281–92.
2. Tonigan JS, Bogenschutz MP, Miller WR. Is alcoholism typology a predictor of both Alcoholics Anonymous affiliation and disaffiliation after treatment? J Subst Abuse Treat 2006;30(4):323–30.
3. Dawson DA, Grant BF, Stinson FS, et al. Estimating the effect of help-seeking on achieving recovery from alcohol dependence. Addiction 2006;101(6):824–34.
4. Narrow WE, Regier DA, Rae DS, et al. Use of services by persons with mental and addictive disorders. Findings from the National Institute of Mental Health Epidemiologic Catchment Area Program. Arch Gen Psychiatry 1993;50(2):95–107.
5. McCrady BS, Epstein EE, Hirsch LS. Issues in the implementation of a randomized clinical trial that includes Alcoholics Anonymous: studying AA-related behaviors during treatment. J Stud Alcohol 1996;57(6):604–12.
6. Morgenstern J, Kahler CW, Frey RM, et al. Modeling therapeutic response to 12-step treatment: optimal responders, nonresponders, and partial responders. J Subst Abuse 1996;8(1):45–59.
7. Humphreys K, Moos RH, Finney JW. Two pathways out of drinking problems without professional treatment. Addict Behav 1995;20(4):427–41.
8. Kaskutas LA, Ammon L, Delucchi K, et al. Alcoholics anonymous careers: patterns of AA involvement five years after treatment entry. Alcohol Clin Exp Res 2005;29(11):1983–90.
9. Humphreys K. Clinicians' referral and matching of substance abuse patients to self-help groups after treatment. Psychiatr Serv 1997;48(11):1445–9.
10. Tonigan JS, Miller WR, Schermer C. Atheists, agnostics and Alcoholics Anonymous. J Stud Alcohol 2002;63(5):534–41.
11. Bogenschutz MP. 12-step approaches for the dually diagnosed: mechanisms of change. Alcohol Clin Exp Res 2007;31(10 Suppl):64s–6s.
12. Tomasson K, Vaglum P. Psychiatric co-morbidity and aftercare among alcoholics: a prospective study of a nationwide representative sample. Addiction 1998;93(3): 423–31.

13. Jordan LC, Davidson WS, Herman SE, et al. Involvement in 12-step programs among persons with dual diagnoses. Psychiatr Serv 2002;53(7):894–6.
14. Tonigan JS. Effectiveness and outcome research. Introduction. Recent Dev Alcohol 2008;18:349–55.
15. Tonigan JS. Alcoholics anonymous outcomes and benefits. Recent Dev Alcohol 2008;18:357–72.
16. Schuckit MA, Tipp JE, Smith TL, et al. Periods of abstinence following the onset of alcohol dependence in 1853 men and women. J Stud Alcohol 1997;58(6):581–9.
17. Gossop M, Stewart D, Marsden J. Attendance at Narcotics Anonymous and Alcoholics Anonymous meetings, frequency of attendance and substance use outcomes after residential treatment for drug dependence: a 5-year follow-up study. Addiction 2008;103(1):119–25.
18. McKellar J, Stewart E, Humphreys K. Alcoholics anonymous involvement and positive alcohol-related outcomes: cause, consequence, or just a correlate? A prospective 2-year study of 2319 alcohol-dependent men. J Consult Clin Psychol 2003;71(2):302–8.
19. McKellar JD, Harris AH, Moos RH. Patients' abstinence status affects the benefits of 12-step self-help group participation on substance use disorder outcomes. Drug Alcohol Depend 2009;99(1–3):115–22.
20. Emrick CD. Alcoholics Anonymous: membership characteristics and effectiveness as treatment. Recent Dev Alcohol 1989;7:37–53.
21. Montgomery HA, Miller WR, Tonigan JS. Does Alcoholics Anonymous involvement predict treatment outcome? J Subst Abuse Treat 1995;12(4):241–6.
22. Tonigan JS. Project Match treatment participation and outcome by self-reported ethnicity. Alcohol Clin Exp Res 2003;27(8):1340–4.
23. Pagano ME, Friend KB, Tonigan JS, et al. Helping other alcoholics in alcoholics anonymous and drinking outcomes: findings from project MATCH. J Stud Alcohol 2004;65(6):766–73.
24. Witbrodt J, Kaskutas LA. Does diagnosis matter? Differential effects of 12-step participation and social networks on abstinence. Am J Drug Alcohol Abuse 2005;31(4):685–707.
25. Kaskutas LA, Bond J, Humphreys K. Social networks as mediators of the effect of Alcoholics Anonymous. Addiction 2002;97(7):891–900.
26. Christo G, Franey C. Drug users' spiritual beliefs, locus of control and the disease concept in relation to Narcotics Anonymous attendance and six-month outcomes. Drug Alcohol Depend 1995;38(1):51–6.

Index

Note: Page numbers of article titles are in **boldface** type.

Prim Care Clin Office Pract 38 (2011) 149–157
doi:10.1016/S0095-4543(11)00009-1
0095-4543/11/$ – see front matter © 2011 Elsevier Inc. All rights reserved.

primarycare.theclinics.com